S0-DCJ-214

MATERNITY MASSAGE

A Healthy Indulgence
A Welcome Relief

Danl Giles, R.N.
Certified Massage Therapist
Independent Wellness Consultant
678-352-0000

MATERNITY MASSAGE

A Healthy Indulgence
A Welcome Relief

BY
CONNIE A. COX

Stress Less Publishing, Inc.
Scottsdale, Arizona

Published in the United States by Stress Less Publishing, Inc.
Copyright ©1994 by Stress Less Publishing, Inc.

All rights reserved. No part of this book may be reproduced or
transmitted in any form or by any means, electronic or
mechanical, including photocopying, recording or by any
information storage and retrieval system, without permission in
writing from the Publisher.

Stress Less Publishing, Inc.
7000 East Camelback Road
Scottsdale, AZ 85251

Library of Congress Cataloging in Publication Data

Cox, Connie A.
Maternity massage : a healthy indulgence, a welcome rellief /by
Connie A. Cox.
    p. cm.
    Includes index
Preassigned LCCN: 94-66358
ISBN   1-885044-01-1

1. Prenatal care. 2. Massage. 3. Pregnancy. I. Title.

RG526.C69 1994   618.2'4
                                        QBI94-1865

Manufactured in the United States of America
First Edition: January, 1994
10 9 8 7 6 5 4 3 2

Photographs by Steve Thompson & Robert Milazzo

Preface

I never thought much about writing a book on maternity massage until 1990. That year someone very close to me who lived in the Midwest surprisingly became pregnant for the first time at the age of 45. Being a regular massage receiver, she never considered changing two massage appointments she had previously made or telling anyone about her pregnancy. She was experimenting with massage, and the pregnancy was her special secret. The first appointment was with someone she was told was very aggressive. The other appointment was with a specialist on shoulders. Her shoulders ached and she needed the relief.

During the first massage, as the woman worked very deeply in the sacral area, she recognized the mistake she had made. She told the woman to stop. She felt somewhat disoriented and queasy afterwards, but she thought she was okay. It was during the shoulder work the next morning that the miscarriage became full-blown. Although she was disappointed to lose the baby, she was more irritated that <u>she</u> had been so stupid about massage and the impact on her pregnancy.

After she woke me at midnight to tell me of her mistake, I became determined to educate women about maternity massage. Massage can be so beneficial to a pregnancy -- it provides one of the few ways to relieve many discomforts of pregnancy. But, a pregnant woman must be an educated consumer. <u>Maternity massage is different</u>. To be most beneficial, it must also change as a pregnancy progresses.

This book was written to clearly explain what a maternity massage should be -- all the nuances -- what to expect. Most important, it presents the information a woman needs to obtain the massage that will be most beneficial for her and her baby.

ACKNOWLEDGMENTS

I greatly appreciate the time and expertise given so freely by the staff of The Stress Less Step who work diligently to insure that every pregnant woman receives just the massage or bodywork that she needs . . .

> Simone Carbone
> Leslie DeNunzio
> Hilda Franco
> Geraldine Kelly
> Marilyn Lavender
> Ofra Naim
> Rebecca Scott
> Pieter Sommen
> Renata Stachowicz-Cebula

I especially want to thank Hilda Franco who is truly *the expert* in maternity massage in the United States. Her knowledge based on twenty years of experience in maternity massage cannot be equaled. Not only did Ms. Franco develop the format and guidelines for practitioners of maternity massage at The Stress Less Step, she has been responsible for maintaining the outstanding quality of maternity massage that has continued. Without Ms. Franco's extensive knowledge and experience this book could not have been written. Nor would so many mothers know the miraculous results of maternity massage.

I also want to express my gratitude to Averill Rider, our model, for her extra patience and willingness to endure whatever we requested -- particularly posing by an ice-cold lake and being chilled to the bone on a mountain cliff.

Lastly, I am very grateful to Dr. Rostilav Tourtchaninov. His critique made such a difference. In addition, he spent the many hours needed to explain anatomical terminology and to teach me the medical aspects of massage.

Table of Contents

INTRODUCTION

Today, more and more women are turning to maternity massage to cope with the physical changes and problems of their pregnancy. They are seeking help with morning sickness, headaches, sinus congestion, back and shoulder pain, swollen legs and feet, and fatigue to name just a few problems. What they are finding is relief! Let me share with you a few experiences of customers of The Stress Less Step . . .

> Jeanette never knew her back could ache so much. The increasing weight of the baby was making her back feel like that of an old woman. She just couldn't move without pain, and she couldn't find a comfortable position for sitting or sleeping. She never thought the gentle massage on her back would help, but what a relief! Her weekly back massages became a necessity for her to enjoy her pregnancy.

> An exhausted Debra needed a solution for insomnia. She was sleeping only a few hours a night, but she still had to work a full day afterwards. Luckily in her sixth month, a friend recommended massage. At the beginning, she found that after each massage she could sleep soundly for about 3 hours. As she continued, she and her baby relaxed even more and she was able to sleep longer each night.

Angela knew that her constant rushing was upsetting the baby. His kicking was very fast and angry, and as she became more stressed, the kicks were faster and harder. She knew she would never stop rushing, that was just the way she had always been. But, she needed something to calm the baby. The answer came during her first massage. The baby settled into a peaceful state with gentle moves and playful kicking. The other surprise came after several more massages: Angela herself became calmer and stopped much of the rushing. She decided then that weekly massages must become a permanent part of her life.

As a rapidly rising corporate star, Marci didn't want her pregnancy to disrupt her career path too much, but she found those difficult and demanding days at work more draining than before. Her solution was a noontime massage. "Going back to work never felt this good." Not only did the massage rejuvenate and energize her, she also found she was more productive and creative once she and the baby were relieved of all the stress of the morning. "I'm ready for anything!"

Every pregnant woman is aware of the many discomforts of pregnancy. As the blood flow accelerates, estrogen increases, and more oxygen is required, many women feel discomfort. They experience "hot flashes," and become irritable, depressed and fearful of the unknown. The baby's increasing weight strains muscles both front and back from the neck all the way down to the toes.

Throughout, the mother's body must stretch more and more to accommodate a growing baby.

These trying physical changes are not the only problems. There are psychological pressures as well. For many women, this is a new experience, and it can be frightening. Not knowing what's really going on inside your body, and hearing all the horror stories of deliveries tests even the most serene new mother. And, the unknowns don't disappear when it's not a first baby. Then, a woman has to cope with both the new baby and the unpredictable behavior of the other children at home.

The result: there is no escaping the tremendous stress and strain of pregnancy. Unfortunately, few remedies or solutions are available for these discomforts and tension. Most medications, tranquilizers, and strenuous exercise are prohibited. Few activities or alternatives offer any reasonable relief.

Fortunately, a maternity massage can safely, comfortably, and effectively relieve much of the increased stress and physical discomforts you will face during your pregnancy. Not only is massage one of the few acceptable and healthy ways to deal with the strains and stresses of pregnancy, it's one of the few pleasures allowed. You may not be able to relax with a glass of wine, but you can get a pampering massage to lessen the pressures, to minimize the strains and stresses, and to eliminate many problems. Don't wait until just before the baby is due to experience the magic of massage. One expectant mother after another who has waited until their eighth or ninth month has said emphatically, "I wish I had done this from the beginning."

As effective and enjoyable as maternity massage may be, few Americans have experienced the benefits and relief. Since the early 1900's, maternity massage has been limited to a handful of experienced practitioners who were taught informally through their own experience or by other massage therapists. Knowledge of maternity massage was literally passed from one massage therapist to another, and because massage was generally considered unacceptable in the United States, this circle of knowledge remained very small. It has only been in the past five years that massage in general has become respectable and more popular. But still, the knowledge and skill regarding maternity massage continue to be limited to a very few practitioners. The pattern of passing knowledge from one massage therapist to another is the primary form of education. It was only 3 to 4 years ago that the first formal training in maternity massage appeared. Even today, training in maternity massage is not required for a massage license, and it is offered in only a small number of massage schools in the United States.

This book tells you what you need to know about maternity massage so that you can reap all of the benefits and enjoy a healthy and serene pregnancy. It reflects the considerable knowledge, experience and skill of the practitioners of maternity massage at The Stress Less Step in New York City and Scottsdale, Arizona.

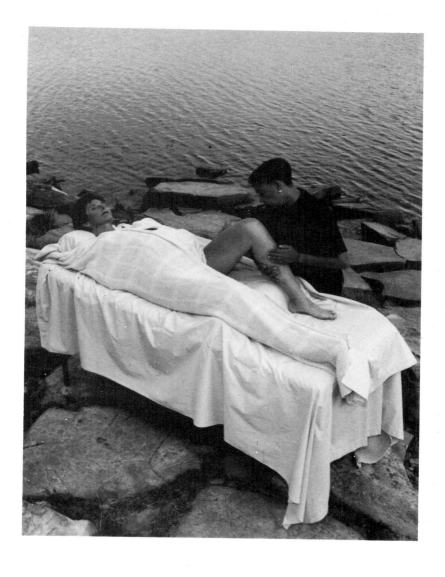

WHY THINK ABOUT A MATERNITY MASSAGE?

Maternity massage is an hour where you will feel pampered and taken care of, but massage offers visible physical benefits that cannot be denied. And you need these benefits for a healthy and enjoyable pregnancy. Most important, the massage will give you more energy and less fatigue. This will be especially clear during the first trimester when fatigue is a prominent complaint. Later in your pregnancy, you will find it difficult to become sufficiently comfortable to sleep soundly for long periods. It is then that many women turn to massage to sleep deeply for several hours after a massage. The relaxing impact of a massage can also calm an active baby so you can relax further.

Other benefits of maternity massage will change as your pregnancy progresses. During the first trimester, a maternity massage can relieve headaches, help to alleviate morning sickness and nausea, and reduce fatigue. The benefits of maternity massage will shift to alleviating backaches, leg cramps, and sciatic-like pain during your second trimester. The most noticeable benefits during the last three months relate to swelling and insomnia. Throughout your pregnancy, the stimulation of the blood flow will assist in the prevention of anemia, a common ailment of pregnant women.

A maternity massage will also benefit you by relieving overall muscle soreness due to exercise or sitting too much. If you are physically active, a massage releases the lactic acid that builds up in muscles. If your work requires sitting a great deal, pressure is often created in the sciatic nerve area, thus causing strain and soreness in your legs as the baby gains weight. Massage will not only help alleviate the stress caused by sitting too much, but it will also work those inactive muscles by toning them.

Furthermore, a maternity massage will aid in your overall muscle tone and elasticity. This is especially important as the baby grows and your body must change to accommodate this growth. Your hips must widen and the muscles around your abdomen, lower back and shoulder will stretch. Your legs must also support more and more weight. Massage is known for its ability to maintain the flexibility in muscles, ligaments, tendons, and joints you will need as your baby grows. Further, massage will alleviate muscle spasms and leg cramps, indications of reduced flexibility in the legs.

A maternity massage also will enhance your relaxation by sedating the nervous system and soothing frazzled nerves. This can be especially helpful with what may feel like sciatic-nerve pain running from the lower back down to the middle of the back of the legs. For many women, this pain begins in the second trimester as the pelvis extends, especially at the joint of the sacrum and pelvic bone on both sides. The resulting sensation is a burning feeling as if the sciatic nerve is inflamed down the leg or just in the calf. A gentle massage of the back and legs reduces this burning sensation as the muscles around the joints are relaxed.

You may be wondering whether or not you need massage just to relieve tension and some of the aches and pains of pregnancy. The answer is "yes!" There are important medical reasons why maternity massage is essential for a healthy and enjoyable pregnancy.

One primary reason massage has such benefits is that it produces a state of deep relaxation. You must remember that it is muscle tension and stress that decreases the needed nutrient absorption and toxin elimination for healthy cells. So the more you relax, the more the cells of your muscles return to their natural state where they function most effectively and efficiently. Your circulation increases, more nutrients are absorbed by your cells, and your lymphatic system removes excessive toxins. Research has also determined that if you are under significant stress over a prolonged period of time, abnormal levels of toxins and chemicals build up in your blood stream and go through the placenta to your baby. Such toxins and chemicals can potentially cause physical problems for your baby. This research makes it critical for you to remain relaxed as much as possible.

If you must live in a stressful environment, then an alternative way to minimize the buildup of toxins is periodic deep relaxation. Massage is just the thing for such deep relaxation. Remember that a relaxing massage can put you in the Alpha state, the first level of meditation. Research completed by Dr. Harold J. Reilly of Edgar Cayce fame also found a gently, relaxing massage to be equivalent to 4 hours of sleep. The positive impact of such relaxation is immediately apparent. It's the result of this deep relaxation that you have a healthy glow after a massage.

But there is more to why massage produces such benefits. The answer lies in the complexity of your body and how any tactile stimulation influences it. You must remember that a massage not only impacts the areas being massaged, but it also affects your entire body because each specific area of your skin and muscles has receptors that are linked to your central nervous system. Different stimuli such as massage techniques prompt varying messages to be sent by these receptors. Certain massage techniques produce signals that cause the cells of your muscles to absorb nutrients more rapidly. Just rub your skin vigorously and you will feel the heat and see the redness prompted by the increased circulation your rubbing produced. Other massage techniques stimulate the drainage function of the cells of your muscles.

With the proper combination and sequence of massage techniques, a massage increases your blood circulation and lymphatic drainage by stimulating the receptors to send messages to increase nutrient absorption and toxin removal. It is this action that produces the beneficial side effects of massage.

For example, fatigue is reduced when you increase the absorption of oxygen and nutrients by the cells of your muscles. With more oxygen and nutrients, you have more energy. It is the gentle, surface massage that prompts the messages sent by the receptors to increase nutrient absorption and stimulate the blood flow to all areas of the body, including the placenta.

Massages also aid your glandular system, thus stabilizing hormonal levels and making their side effects less severe. Through massage, each gland is stimulated, enhanced, and balanced. One important gland affected by massage is the thyroid gland. During pregnancy, the thyroid gland sometimes goes into over-production. This over-production causes irritability, "hot flashes," increased pulse rates and rapid, short breathing. Through massage, the thyroid gland is maintained and balanced thus decreasing the negative side effects of too much thyroid. Massage also balances an overactive metabolism rate produced by excess thyroid.

Another gland affected by massage is your adrenal gland. Pregnancy increases the adrenal hormone levels. Excessive amounts of these hormones can cause a pinkness in your skin. They are also believed to be one cause of edema. Massage is one of the most effective approaches for relaxing your adrenal glands and reducing the amount of adrenal hormones generated during your pregnancy. Stimulation of your lymphatic drainage system complements this relaxation of your adrenal glands by reducing excess amounts of adrenal hormones.

By stimulating your lymph drainage system, massage may additionally reduce the possibility of brown patches or areas appearing in your skin. Research has indicated that massage may reduce the levels of melanin, the substance responsible for these brown patches. When you are pregnant, your placenta generates hormones that prompt increased production of melanin. If your lymph drainage system is not functioning well, this excessive concentration of melanin in the melanocyte cells of your skin causes brown spots. A better-functioning lymph drainage system resulting from massage is believed to keep the melanin at low enough levels so that brown patches will not occur.

The last important gland effected by massage is your thymus gland. Massage stimulates this gland so that is can help fight off infection by boosting the immune system.

Furthermore, a maternity massage assists your lymphatic system in the removal of toxins from cells. Your lymphatic system is directly related to the condition of the muscles. There is no pump such as the heart for your lymphatic system. Lymph moves freely until muscles tense. When muscles are tensed either by exercise or stress, the lymph movement decreases dramatically and the concentration of toxins rises. To release this buildup, you must relax your muscles and increase lymph drainage. Massage is one of the best ways to stimulate the needed drainage after tension. Regular massage helps keep muscles in a more relaxed state so that buildups do not occur.

Lymphatic drainage is also critical for making your circulation faster and more efficient - a key to good health for you and your baby during your pregnancy. Your lymphatic system removes toxins from cells and your blood stream and produces the white blood cells called lymphocytes in your lymphatic nodes and thymus. With the removal of toxins, your blood can carry more oxygen and nutrients to your cells and tissues. This increases your red blood cell count. Then your cells can regenerate more easily and quickly. Massage assists the effectiveness of your lymph system by stimulating lymph nodes to more efficiently remove toxins from your body. The outward signs of a well-functioning lymph drainage system are more energy, less fatigue, and increased immunity.

An efficient lymphatic system also helps to prevent complications due to excessive toxins. For example, during pregnancy, many women experience varicose veins, an accumulation of toxic wastes in the veins. A massage can control the development of varicose veins by its draining effect and its facilitation of the reduction of swelling in the legs. Toxemia occurs because the lymphatic system ceases to remove toxins from tissues and cells. Massage helps maintain the effective functioning of the lymphatic system.

Without good circulation, well-balanced glandular secretions, and an effective lymph system, the negative side effects of pregnancy such as irritability, depression, fear of the unknown, and hot flashes worsen. It's the combination of relaxation and stimulating messages to

prompts your body to effectively
ur pregnancy as a result of massage.

prepare your muscles for the strain and
Massage adds tone and flexibility to
what your muscles need for the
of labor. So with regular maternity
uscles will be in better condition for the

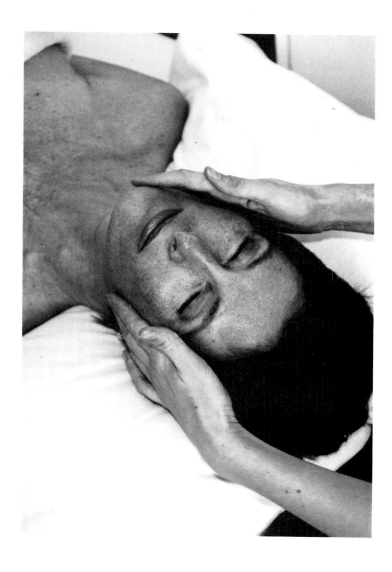

WHAT IS
A MATERNITY MASSAGE?

A maternity massage is a light, pampering massage which increases your circulation and the removal of toxins from your cells and blood stream while producing the necessary level of relaxation throughout your body. The movements and techniques are derived from traditional massage. They have been adapted to meet the specific needs and problems of pregnancy.

Traditional massage was developed as part of ancient folk medicine. The instinctive gesture of rubbing to ease pain was the first step toward massage and sources indicate it was used extensively in Ancient Egypt, Greece, Rome, and China as early as 2700 BC. Even Hippocrates, the father of ancient medicine, wrote, "The physician should be experienced in many things, and no less massage . . ." Today's massage techniques evolved primarily in Sweden, eastern Europe, and Russia, where scientific research was utilized to correctly determine and measure the impact of massage techniques in the treatment and restoration of specific muscle capability, the elimination of fatigue, the maintenance of muscle tone, and the strengthening of health and prevention of disease.

The character of a massage is determined by the massage technique used, the strength of the motion, the tempo of the movements, and the duration of the massage. Techniques such as rubbing and stroking relax the body while digging, vibrating, and striking simulate. A gentle surface massage increases blood circulation and the lymph system, while a deeper massage inhibits these two systems. A rapid massage stimulates the nervous system while a slower massage calms it. And, the longer a massage is performed, the more it relaxes the nervous system. By varying the technique, speed, force, and length of a massage, it is possible to influence the primary systems of your body in many different ways to produce a number of desired results. As Leandr Koshitel, an expert in Russian massage, so clearly pointed out, "The art of massage can be compared with the art of the sculptor, with the exception of the fact that the masseur works with living tissue . . . the art of massage is a gift."

The goal for your maternity massage is to produce a total relaxation of muscles while peacefully stimulating your blood circulation, lymphatic drainage and endocrinological balance. This will not only reduce the stress in your body, it will also settle your emotional state.

To accomplish this, it is necessary for your massage therapist to ensure two conditions are met before your massage can begin. The first condition is placing your body in a position to maximize the complete relaxation of your muscles. This occurs only when your extremities are bent at the joints at desired angles.

To begin a maternity massage, you first lie down on your back. A bolster or pillow will be placed under your knee joints to effectively relax the muscles in your legs . . .

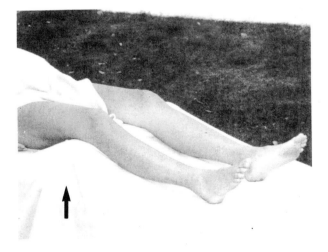

This bolster under your knees will also eliminate any strain in your lower back and abdominal muscles.

Your arms will be bent so that your hands easily rest on your belly or just below your belly on your abdomen . . .

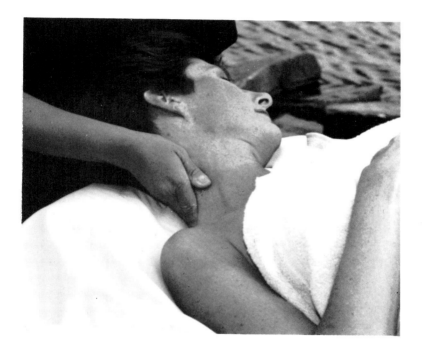

A small pillow will also be placed under your head to relax your neck and its joints. Your head will be elevated slightly more if you are experiencing tension or pain in your diaphragm area.

It is also necessary for the massage therapist to make sure you remain warm throughout the massage. Depending upon the warmth of the room, you may be covered with an additional blanket and/or towels . . .

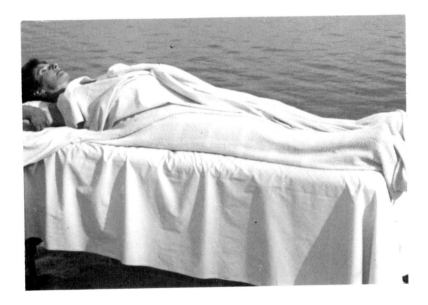

Coolness unfortunately prompts your muscles to tense automatically and this coolness hampers the effectiveness of the massage. Even if the room is warm, you should be covered at least with a towel placed over your torso and positioned between your thighs.

Once you are comfortably positioned and warmly
covered, the massage therapist will stand or sit at your
head for just a couple of moments to orient themselves to
you . . .

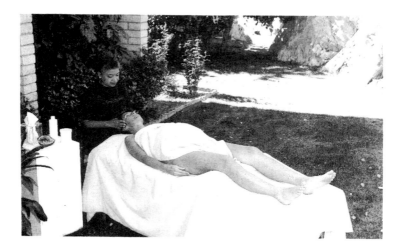

During this time, you can take a few steps to enhance what
you will experience. First take one or two deep breaths all
the way down to your abdomen. If you want, hold your
breath for a count of three and then slowly exhale through
your mouth, or just breathe deeply. After several deep
breaths, let yourself begin to breath very easily and
comfortably. The way you breath naturally is perfect. Let
your mind wander to a favorite place of yours to relax.
Think back to whatever place you remember as a

wonderful place to relax and feel peaceful. Perhaps you love lying in the sun on a beautiful white beach or sitting comfortably by a peaceful stream or waterfall. Whatever your preference, that's the place for your mind to be. Just think of your favorite place and enjoy remembering all the details of why that place is so special -- the sounds, the fragrances, the colors . . . each little detail. From then on, just relax and let the massage therapist do all the work.

A maternity massage starts with your head and face . . .

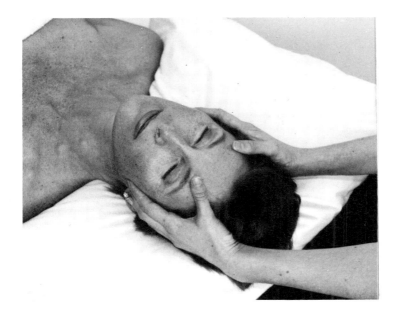

At the beginning of the massage, when the massage therapist is massaging your head, let your body become comfortable with the massage therapist's touch -- the way the person's hands feel as they massage your temples, scalp, and jaws . . .

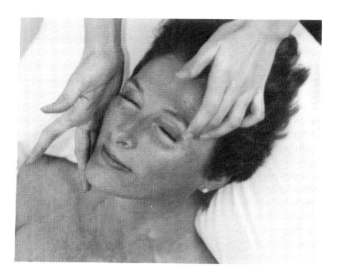

The massage therapist will use calming massage techniques such as gentle strokes as they work on your head. Special attention will be paid to the occipital region -- at the base of the skull in the back. Stimulation of this area will increase the flow of your body's endorphins and enkephalins, your own natural tranquilizers and pain killers. This is very important at the beginning of your massage because these natural tranquilizers will help calm your mind and make you more peaceful. You can then relax sufficiently to experience the pleasure of your body receiving a massage.

Once the massage therapist has massaged your head and senses a increasing state of relaxation in the muscles of your head, they will move to your neck. The massage movement will be downward toward your shoulders. This downward direction is necessary to correctly enhance the lymph drainage from the head to the cluster of lymph nodes in the neck . . .

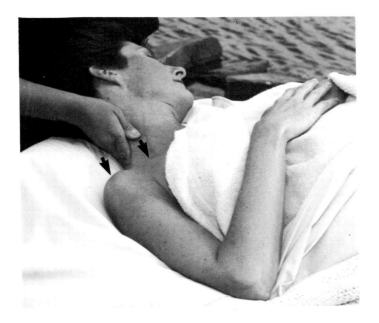

When your neck begins to relax, the massage therapist will shift the massage to your shoulders and chest where most women hold tension and stress.

A combination of strokes and gentle rocking is particularly effective for relaxing tense shoulders. Just pushing slightly downward on your shoulders can begin to bring them into a more relaxed position . .

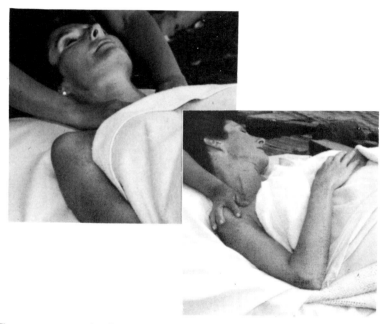

The movement will continue to be downward. This will stimulate your circulation to your heart and lymph movement toward the cluster of lymph nodes near your underarms.

In an hour-long massage, you can expect your massage therapist to spend between 5 to 10 minutes on your head neck, and shoulders.

After your shoulders, come your left hand and left arm. The flow of all massage movements will be from your hand toward your shoulder . . .

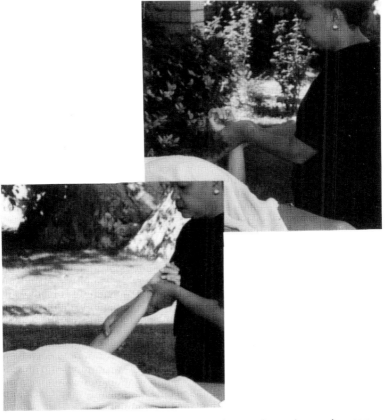

Typically, the massage of each of your hands and arms will continue for about 4 to 5 minutes. This time will be lengthened if your hands become swollen during the later stages of your pregnancy.

Then slowly, the massage therapist will proceed from your left arm and hand to your left foot and leg. Just as on your arm, the work will be done from your feet upward to your hips and torso . . .

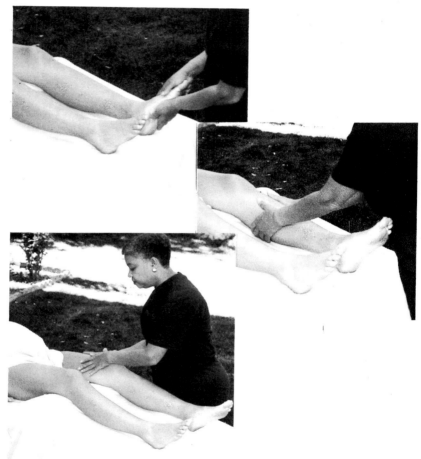

About 8 minutes will be spend on each leg. If you are experiencing swollen feet and ankles, this time will be increased.

Your massage therapist will continue to work clockwise around your body -- to correspond to the natural clockwise flow of your body . . .

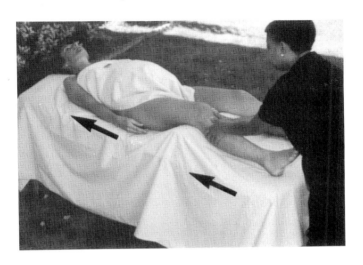

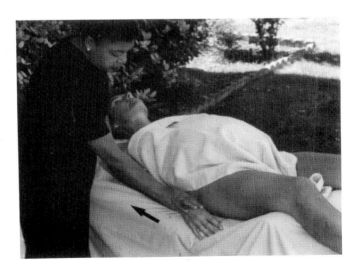

Once the front of your body has been completed, you will be turned so that your back can be massaged . . .

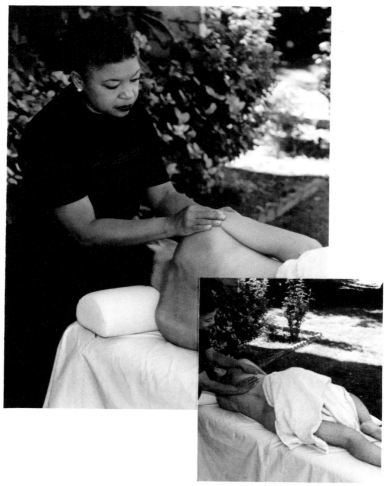

Approximately 20 minutes will be spent on your back. The portion spend on your lower back versus your shoulders will depend upon the location of your muscle tension.

At the end, the massage therapist will have you sit up so that your neck, shoulders and back can be worked from a different position. This sitting position is needed to release any tension remaining in these areas. You will find that your massage therapist will spend about 5 to 8 minutes working with you in this sitting position.

During a maternity massage six different types of massage strokes or techniques will be used. The massage of each body area will begin with long, smooth strokes toward your torso or heart using their whole hand. . .

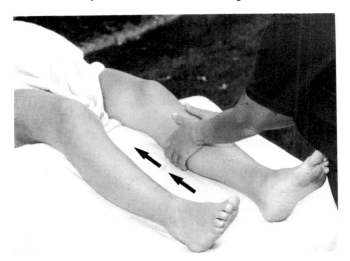

Your massage therapist will be moving their hands so that they mold their hands to the contours of your body. These initial long strokes are very important for several reasons. First, they relax and prepare your muscles for somewhat deeper work. It is also during these long strokes that your massage therapist will be looking for tension. Lastly, these strokes are used to spread the oil on your skin.

After the beginning long strokes, you may notice your massage therapist using the base of their palm to rub over the same area. These longer strokes done with the base of the palm add a little additional pressure and relax your muscles even more.

Once the muscles are ready for stronger techniques, the initial long strokes will be followed by five other massage techniques. My favorite technique is the coil-like motion that is in fact circles being made with the closed middle fingers of your massage therapist's hand. . .

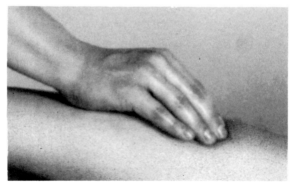

This technique is used in many areas in a maternity massage. It works very well on thinner, smaller muscles like those on the sides of your calves and on your arms.

On the chest area, these circles stimulate lymphatic drainage to your underarm. They will be done from your collar bone or the center of your chest toward your underarm. . . .

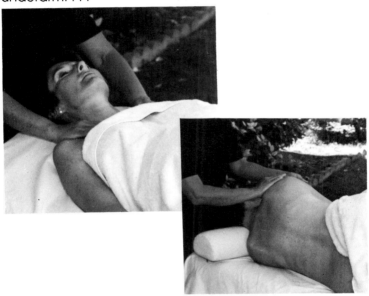

They are also very effective for gently releasing tension in your shoulders as you are lying on your side. A few massage therapists may use these circles on your thighs, but they must have very strong fingers to utilize this technique well on thicker muscles.

Kneading, just like what you do with bread dough, will be used primarily on your hips and legs . . .

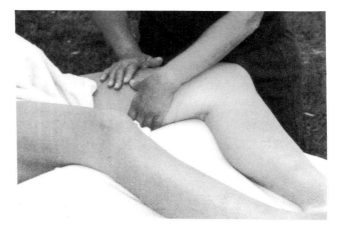

Kneading is very effective for releasing tension in larger, thicker muscles and stimulating circulation in fatty tissue. It is done with a closed hand.

Another technique is a gentle pulling of muscles. It feels like your massage therapist is using alternative hands to rub your muscles with somewhat more strength than you feel with the initial strokes -- so that they are pulled slightly . .

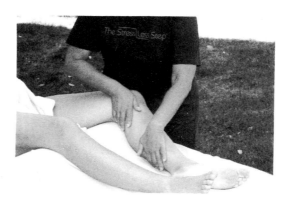

In addition, you will feel your massage therapist rhythmically squeezing your muscles as they move over thicker muscles and fatty tissue. This squeezing is nothing like pinching. It is done in a gentle way with the whole hand.

Lastly, you may find your massage therapist gently vibrating a certain area. This is normally done when other techniques are not effectively releasing tension. Although gentle, vibration is very powerful at relaxing muscles. Few U.S. massage schools teach this technique so you may not encounter it very often.

In a maternity massage, all of the strokes and techniques are applied in the gentle manner that is necessary to stimulate circulation and your lymph system. Remember these systems are only stimulated by gentle strokes, not deep work.

The directions for all the movements and strokes will be towards the heart or major clusters of lymph nodes. Some clusters of lymph nodes are located at the joints of your elbows and knees. The primary clusters of lymph nodes are located in the groin area, in the underarms and the chest right above the underarms, and in the middle of your torso. To most effectively stimulate lymph drainage, massage strokes will generally follow the flow of the lymph toward the nearest lymph nodes, although the lymph nodes will not be massaged. For example, massage of the legs is done toward your hips and abdomen . . .

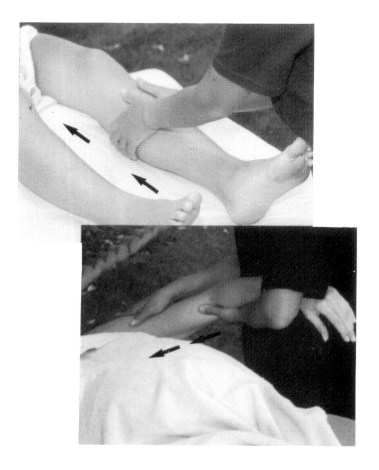

The massage of your shoulders and chest will be toward your underarms. The massage of your arms will be directed to your chest and armpits where critical lymph nodes are located. To facilitate lymph drainage, your arms should be slightly bent at both your elbow and shoulder. Your arms should be raised no more than 4 or 5 inches from the table. If they are raised up at a ninety-degree angle from the shoulder or over your head, the position creates sufficient muscle tension in your arm and shoulder along the lymph flows that it impedes lymphatic drainage. Raising your arm also pulls the muscles of your back and adds unnecessary stress to your back muscles.

The movement toward the heart is what is primarily responsible for the increase in circulation of blood. Keeping the movements matched to lymph flows on relaxed muscles insures the lymphatic drainage is maximized.

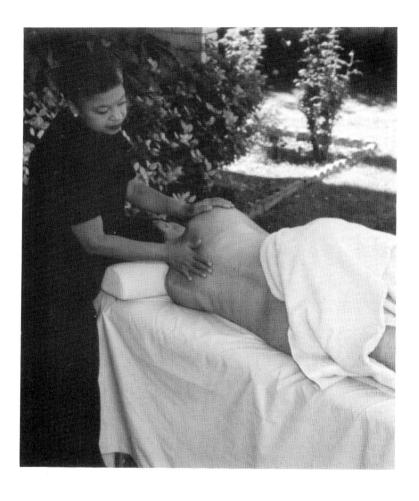

HOW DOES A MATERNITY MASSAGE DIFFER?

Although maternity massage techniques are derived from Swedish massage, you will discover that a maternity massage differs in several critical aspects . . .

- The positions of your body during the massage
- The intensity of the bodywork
- The areas of concentration

You may also notice that the massage therapist uses more oil now that you are pregnant. This is usually the case because your skin becomes drier. Let's look at each of the primary differences so that you'll clearly understand what will happen.

Body Positions

During a maternity massage, the positioning of your body is very important to enhance your comfort and reduce any strain in your muscles. Every effort should be taken to minimize any muscle discomfort and to not hinder circulation. Only when a pregnant women is comfortable can an effective massage be given.

During the first and second trimester, a pregnant woman can still lie on her back easily and comfortably for a fairly long period. And, most of the massage is completed with her lying on her back during the first trimester. To insure that stomach, back & shoulder muscles are sufficiently relaxed so that an effective massage can be done, your knees are bent and a bolster or pillow is placed underneath them for support . . .

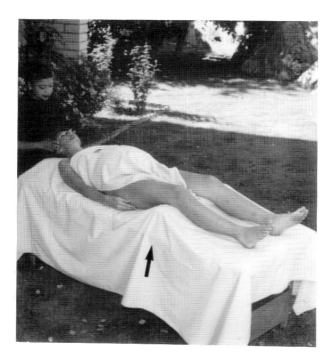

Also, a small pillow is placed under your head, neck and shoulders . . .

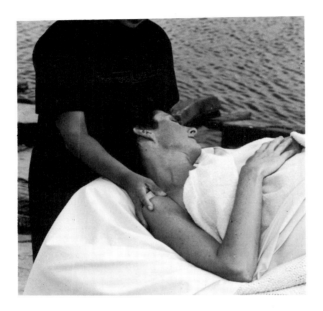

This results in the neck bending slightly forward so that the muscles of the stomach and shoulders can relax further. You will find that the placement of this pillow under the neck and shoulders also makes breathing much easier because it takes the strain from the diaphragm that is caused by larger breasts and an expanding belly.

To massage the back of the woman's body, the woman lies on her side . . .

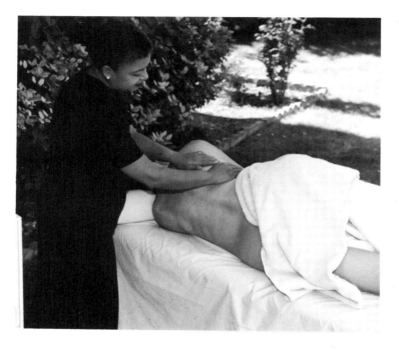

To position a woman correctly, the spine must be kept as straight as possible and the woman's body must be stable so that it does not move substantially when massage strokes are applied.

To accomplish these two goals, the bottom leg is placed on a straight line as a continuation of the spine and the top leg is bent . . .

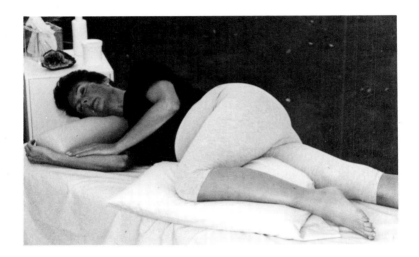

A pillow is then placed between the legs and underneath the knee of the bent leg . . .

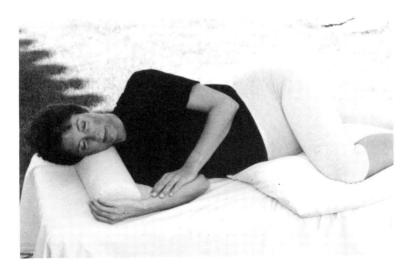

Another pillow may be placed by and slightly under your waist and slightly under your belly or the pillow underneath your leg may be moved so that this pillow is also under your waist . . .

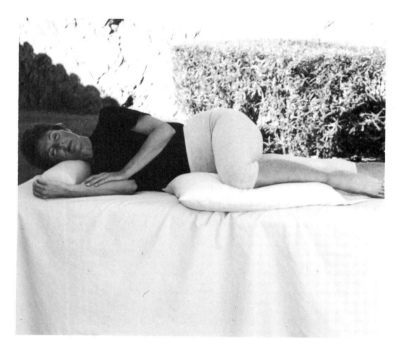

Lastly, a neck roll is placed between the shoulders and head.

It is this key position that keeps a pregnant woman and her baby in a comfortable position with no pressure on the back, stomach, neck or spine.

You will find this placement of pillows puts you in one of the most comfortable positions of all. This position is so comfortable that many pregnant women use the same position and placement of pillows to sleep peacefully at home.

Once you have entered your last trimester, most of the massage will be completed with you lying on your sides. The amount of time you lie on your back will depend on the position of your baby and any discomfort you feel.

Bodywork Intensity

Another obvious difference of a maternity massage is the intensity of the work. A maternity massage must always be gentle and relaxing. This is especially true during the first trimester when the embryo is most unstable. No one is really sure what can dislodge the embryo and result in a miscarriage during this period. Most experts believe that dramatic changes are the culprit. That is why extra caution is required during a massage given in the first trimester. A capable massage therapist knows that most miscarriages occur during the first trimester and they will avoid all potential disruptions. The massage can be done a little stronger as the pregnancy enters the third trimester.

A gentle massage is necessary for other reasons. Your heart rate and blood pressure escalate rapidly if any pain is generated during a massage. Such rapid increases in blood pressure and heart rates are not good for your baby. Instead, your baby needs stable blood pressure and a constant heart rate, just what a gentle, relaxing massage will produce. In addition, when your body is working as hard as a pregnancy demands, your body's adrenaline is substantially below normal levels and your body becomes somewhat defenseless. At this time, your body is not able to cope well with physical afflictions. The result is that a problem might be caused by an improper or too strong massage.

Most important is the negative impact a stronger massage may have on your baby. The baby inside of you is most comfortable when it feels gentle, rhythmic motion, like when you are walking easily. Your baby will be most uncomfortable with sudden or strong changes and movements. Scientific research has even shown that your baby will respond dramatically when it feels such discomfort. A strong, vigorous massage will produce the dramatic and sudden changes in your internal environment that can prompt unpleasant and vigorous responses from your baby.

During a maternity massage, it is important that you never feel the massage therapist digging into a muscle with a finger or thumb . . .

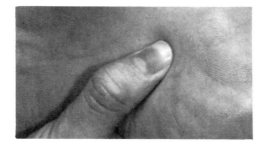

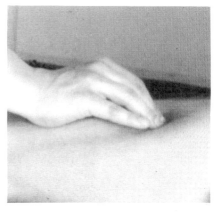

<u>No Digging With Fingertips</u>

One massage therapist says that if you feel a massage therapist use a single finger or knuckles instead of the broad part of their hand or palm, you should stop the massage immediately. Only with the whole hand or palm can massage techniques be done without any potential negative impact on you or your baby.

Don't worry about a light, gentle massage not having any impact. Even with strokes applied in a gentle manner, you will experience all the benefits of massage. Blood-flow and lymphatic drainage are stimulated by the lightest pressure, not deep work. A lymph drainage massage in fact is one of the lightest massages of all, no matter on whom it is done, man or woman. Gently massaging the sciatic nerve area also relieves any inflammation and pain a pregnant woman may be experiencing. A maternity massage is one situation where gentleness and tenderness produce the best results.

Areas of Concentration

There are a number of areas on your body where there will be a noticeable shift in time spent. You will find certain areas will be given much more time and attention now that you are pregnant. To maintain your circulation, more time is needed on your extremities such as your hands and feet. You will find your arms being stroked upward to remove excess fluid and toxins. And, the massage of your legs will be upward from the foot to the thigh so that your lymph will flow toward the lymph nodes in the groin area. This procedure helps this important lymphatic area cleanse and remove excess fluid and toxins from your legs.

Because your legs and feet are working harder with the increasing weight, a capable massage therapist will spend much more time to eliminate the fatigue and overwork in your legs and feet . . .

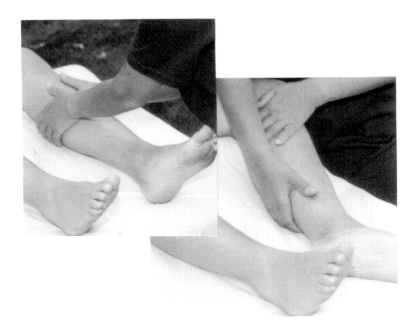

Many massage therapists will also spend more time on your thighs where stretch marks tend to occur . . .

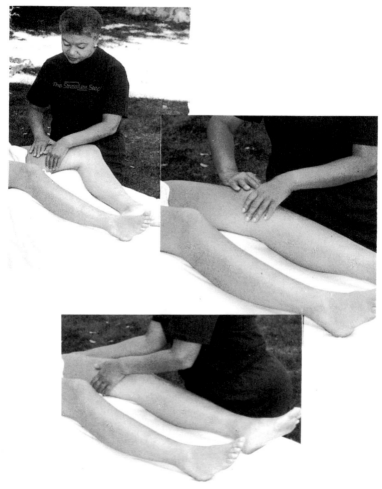

Frequent and effective massage is believed to minimize these marks by maintaining a high level of flexibility and elasticity of the skin in these areas.

There are a number of areas on your body where there will be a noticeable reduction of time and attention. In a regular massage, more time is spent on both men and women on the neck, shoulders, and lower back. This is where a majority of people carry muscle tension. Unfortunately, many pregnant women demand more time and firmness on their shoulders and lower back, but it is precisely these areas which are avoided during a maternity massage.

Why are these areas so important for a maternity massage. First, the lower back on the left side is where the placenta is connected to your body . . .

<u>Critical Area for Very Gentle Massage</u>

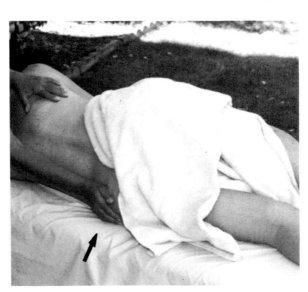

If too much pressure is applied in this area, it can potentially break a weak placenta connection.

The other areas that are avoided relate to meridian points on energy flows that are connected to the vagina and cervix. Over stimulation of these points during a massage can cause the vagina to relax, the cervix to open, and the embryo to be discharged. These points are located . . .

1. Between the ankle and Achilles tendon

<u>An Area to be Avoided</u>

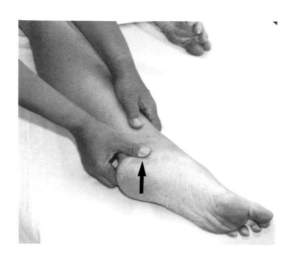

2. Five inches up from the ankle on the
   inside of the calf

   ### An Area to Be Avoided

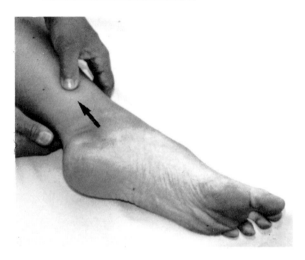

3. In the fleshy part between the index finger
   and the thumb

   ### An Area for Minimal Pressure

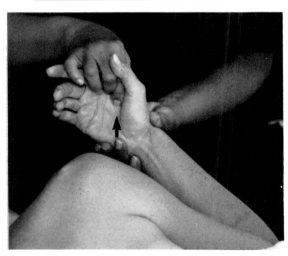

Because stimulation of these points prompts the vagina to relax, the cervix to open and the baby to move, it is exactly these points and places that are worked on during labor to speed up the delivery process, as you will see in the chapter "Shiatsu for Labor."

There are several additional places where only a careful, delicate massage can be done. These areas include . . .

1. Along the neck & collar-bone area

The Area for Delicate Massage

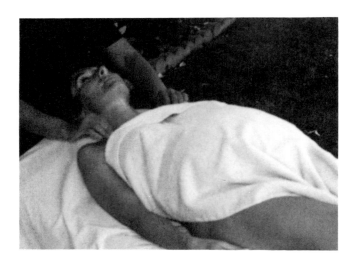

2. Around the shoulder blades

An Area for Delicate Massage

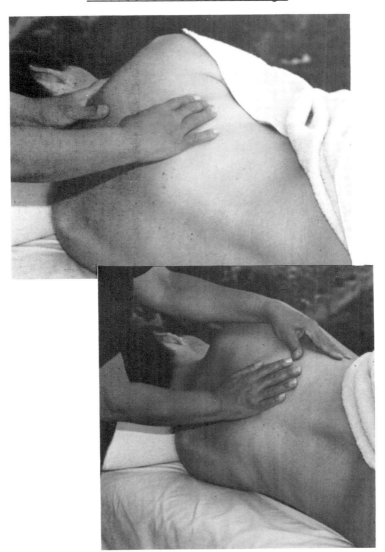

3. Near the sacrum (lower back)

An Area for Delicate Massage

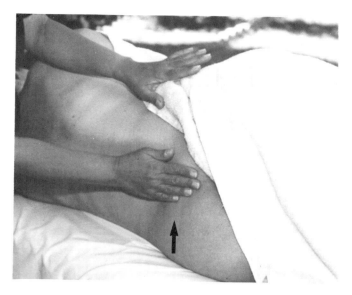

Besides the possibility of a miscarriage, over stimulation of these points can result in bleeding, spotting, mild contractions, premature labor, and a shift in the position of the baby. Too much pressure and too much time spent working these points can also produce the opening or dilating of the cervix.

An additional area where a massage therapist will use caution is around the knees . .

An Area for Very Gentle Massage

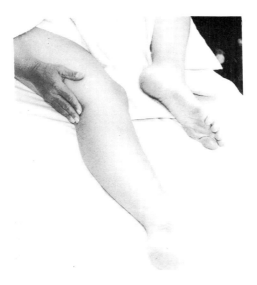

This area around the knees is important because of varicose veins. Not only will varicose veins be completely avoided, but the area is massaged gently so as not to aggravate any problematic conditions.

Lastly, your belly should never be massaged by anyone but you, a midwife or your doctor. There are just too many unknowns, potential problems and insufficient benefits for this area to be massaged. More important, babies can change positions when a mother's belly is massaged. You may find your doctor massaging your belly just before amniocentesis to move the baby out of the way. Because of all the unknowns about pregnancy, there may be other minor problems or conditions that could be aggravated by the belly being massaged. A capable massage therapist will exercise caution especially since there are no known benefits to be gained by massaging the belly. Remember the muscle strain occurs on the muscles surrounding the belly, not on the belly itself. Massaging the muscles surrounding the belly will reduce the strain. So, there is little to justify your belly being rubbed during a maternity massage.

DON'T FORGET REFLEXOLOGY !

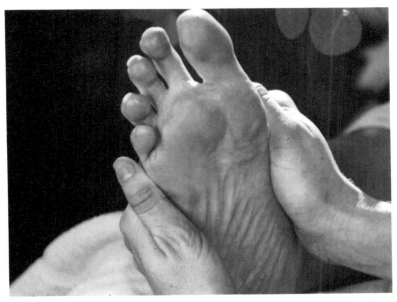

You may find that one of your favorite parts of a maternity massage is when your feet are being rubbed. With the added weight of the baby, your feet are doing so much more. If this is the case, you should experiment with reflexology. Reflexology is not just a foot massage, it is an ancient healing art which is performed on the feet. A typical reflexology session begins with a foot massage to relax your feet. It is followed by pressure being applied evenly primarily on the bottom of your feet. This ancient healing art can be very helpful when you are pregnant.

You can also learn how to do it on yourself during the first months to relieve morning sickness and fatigue. Here's how it works and what you can do.

Today's reflexology is based on research conducted by Eunice Ingham, based on the zone therapy of Dr. William Fitzgerald. Dr. Fitzgerald discovered that the systems of your body work in zones that run lengthwise from your head to your toes. There are ten zones, five on each side of your body. These same zones are in your hands and feet . . .

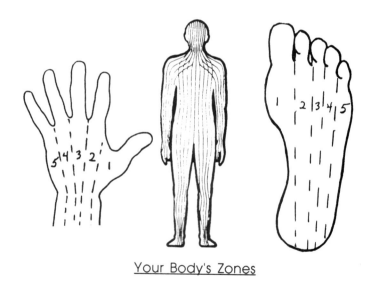

Your Body's Zones

When you change something in one location of your body, you impact the systems in the entire zone. For example, if you want to eliminate pain in one place, you only need to apply pressure in a corresponding place within the zone. For excellent physical health, all of the systems in your body such as circulation and lymph drainage must flow evenly and easily. Periodically, these flows and systems need to be balanced and revitalized.

Ms. Ingham found that you could access these systems via your nervous system by applying pressure on the feet and hands, very sensitive and accessible places. Not only are your body's systems and flows mirrored in your feet; organs, glands, and body parts are connected to corresponding areas of the foot . . .

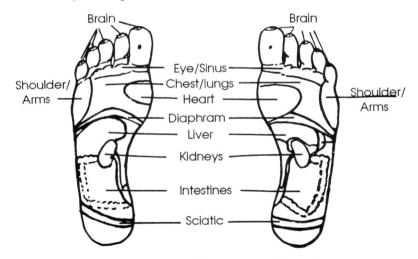

Your Feet as Minimaps of Your Body

Reflexologists have found that your feet respond as if your feet and hands are minimaps of your body.

By applying pressure to appropriate points on your feet, you can break down blocks and balance flows in other parts of your body. You gain homeostasis. Reflexology can also improve your circulation, stimulate your body's natural healing abilities, and eliminate stress and tension.

Reflexology for pregnant women differs from standard reflexology sessions in many of the same ways that a maternity massage differs from a regular massage. Most important, reflexology for pregnancy is a gentle reflexology session. This gentleness is needed so that the impact on your baby is not overwhelming. Normally, the session will begin with a massage of your feet . . .

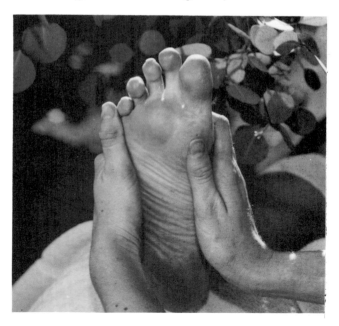

This massage relaxes your feet and prepares them for pressure point work on your reflex points.

Pressure point work will be completed initially in a very systematic way. The reflexologist will begin to apply pressure along points on your heel and then work upwards. Some reflexologists work across your foot and then gradually work upwards . . .

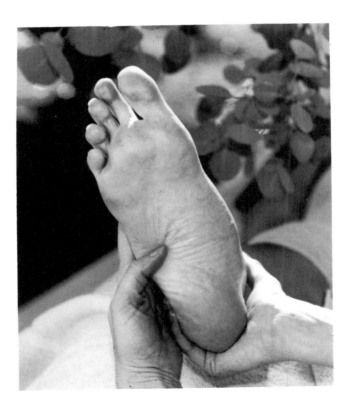

Others will work on a line from the bottom of your heel to up to your toes.

As your reflexologist applies pressure, you may feel some minor pain in a few areas. For example, all people are sensitive on the reflex point for the pituitary gland located in the big toe. . .

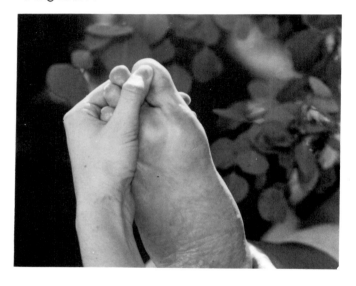

Many people are also sensitive on the points related to the adrenal glands.

You may also feel some discomfort when the reflexologist encounters a problem, such as an upset stomach. Otherwise, the session should be very, very enjoyable. It is important to remember that the pressure used by the reflexologist should be sufficient to make changes, but not great enough to provoke pain.

In addition, there are reflexology points that will be avoided while you are pregnant. These points relate to your reproductive system. These points are located below the ankle on the inside and outside of the foot . . .

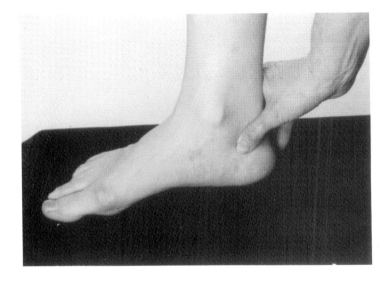

Inappropriate pressure on these points can induce labor, provoke cramps or create a greater, heavier stress level in your body.

Lastly, pressure on the solar plexus will be minimal. This area is located right in the center of your foot, just beside the ball of your foot . . .

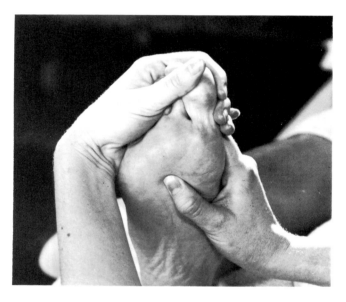

You may find reflexology to be just what you need for many of the discomforts of pregnancy. Most women fall asleep immediately during reflexology sessions . . . its relaxation impact is that quick and that powerful. Also, working through your feet and hands is a safe and effective way to work on specific areas of your body without direct physical contact with those areas impacting your womb. For example, much of the strain and pressure on your spine can be relieved by working the arch of your foot. There is no need to apply deep pressure on your back and the area where the placenta is connected. Or, your stomach can be accessed without any physical contact with your belly and your baby. The reflexologist just works on the middle area of the sole of your foot.

Reflexology is worth a try no matter how skeptical you may be of its philosophy and beneficial claims. At the least, your lymph drainage and circulation will be stimulated so that the swelling in your feet and hands will be less. The most that can happen is that you will feel fantastic after each session -- the nausea will lessen, the aches and pains will be relieved, and your energy will be renewed.

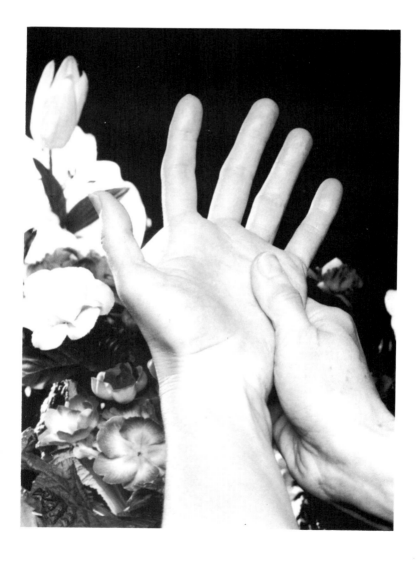

REFLEXOLOGY YOU CAN DO YOURSELF

The best part of reflexology is that you can do it yourself.
At the beginning of your pregnancy, you may want to do it
on your feet. As you progress, it will be easier to do
reflexology on your hands . . .

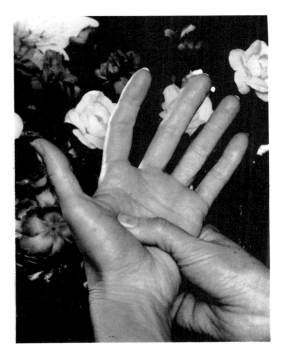

If you are right-handed, work first on your left hand and then
switch to your right hand. If you are left-handed, start
working on your right hand.

Morning sickness

To alleviate nausea, the best place to work is the pituitary gland. This is located on the thumb at the center of the spiral or loop . . .

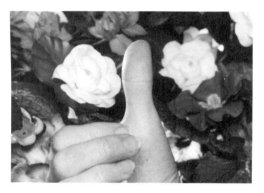

You should use the tip of the thumb of your opposite hand to push on this point. Then as you are pushing on this point, move your thumb back toward your fingers . . .

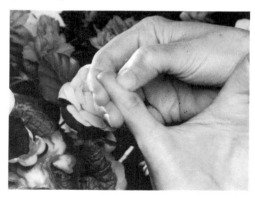

Repeat this pressure just a few times on each thumb. If you feel a little pain, don't be surprised. The pituitary gland is very sensitive.

You can also work the diaphragm area on your palms to help reduce morning sickness. The diagram area is located below the knuckles on the inside of the palm . . .

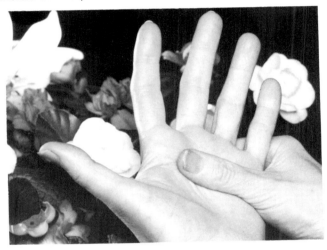

To work this area, you will let your thumb move across this area in what I call 'an inch-worm' movement. Reflexologists call this "walking." Place the back of your thumb on the edge of your hand, then bend your thumb at the first knuckle . . .

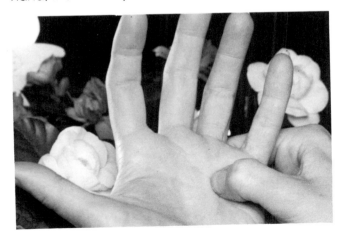

Next, straighten your thumb . . .

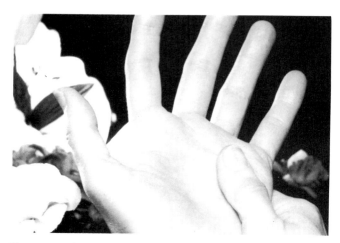

Then apply some pressure at this new place by bending your thumb again at the first knuckle. . .

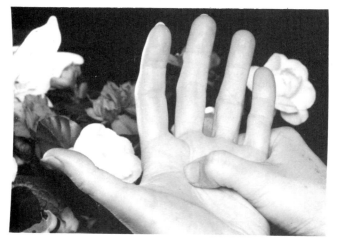

Keep bending your thumb at the first knuckle and straightening it and move across the back of your hand in the diaphragm area. Let your thumb continue to inch back and forth across this area.

The last approach for relieving morning sickness involves applying pressure on the tip of all your fingers and thumb with a finger or thumb of your opposite hand . . .

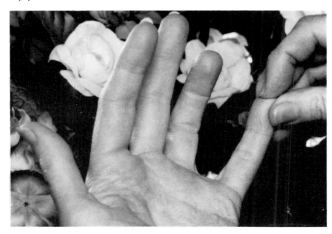

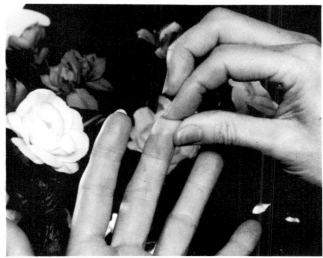

This pressure helps relax your nervous system and therefore your body's reaction to the changes that are producing the morning sickness.

Swollen Legs, Ankles and Feet

The best way to alleviate swelling is to stimulate
your lymph system. To do this, you want to work the
wrist area of each hand. First, hold your forearm a
couple of inches above your wrist . .

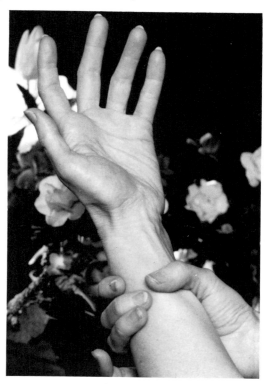

Then rub your arm down to your hand. Do this a
couple of times on each wrists.

Then make a fist with one hand and use the other hand to gently and slowly rotate your fist two or three times to the right . . .

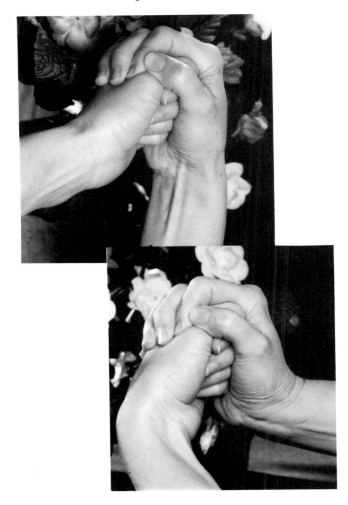

and then two or three times to the left. After that, change hands.

Open your hand and use your thumb to gently rub across the palms of each hand. The motion should be like a windshield wiper going only in one direction . . .

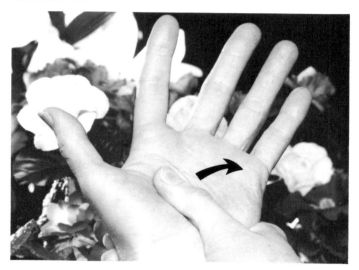

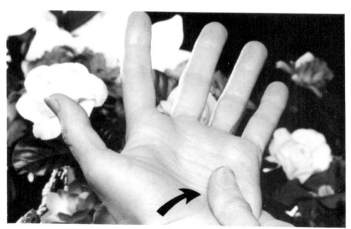

That is, wipe your thumb toward the fingers of your second hand. Let your thumb start at the wrist and work up to the fingers.

Lastly, turn your hand over so that you are looking at the top of your hand. Gently rub your thumb along the path from the bottom of each finger at the wrist to its tip alongside the bone . . .

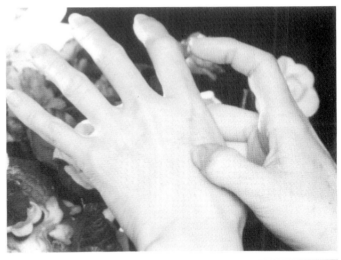

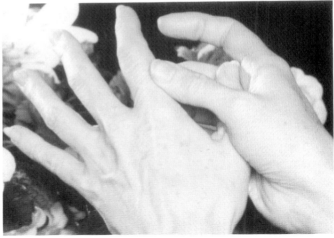

You want to apply pressure in the space between the bones and along the outside of each finger. These are the lymph drainage areas.

Fatigue

There are several ways to eliminate fatigue. First, you need to work the area below the knuckle line on the palm of your hand, the same area worked for nausea. To work this area, hold your hand flat and let your thumb inch-worm or "walk" its way across this area as you did for morning sickness. Then loosen the hand being worked and as you inch-worm or walk across the same area, let your fingers flex as you apply pressure . . .

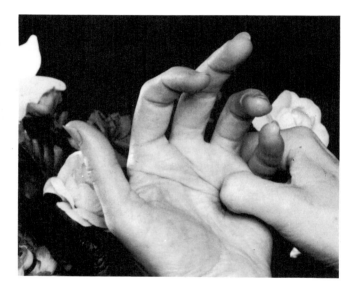

That is, push so that each finger flops down into a hanging position.

Back pain

For relief of back pain, "inch-worm" or walk your thumb in small steps all along the outside edge of your hand, from below the pinkie finger to the top of the wrist, and then from the top of the thumb to the wrist.

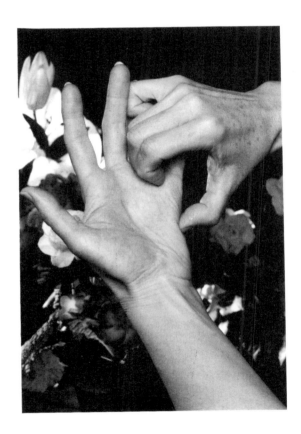

Spend a little more time in the area below the wrist.
In addition, you should also focus on the area
below the knuckle on both sides . . .

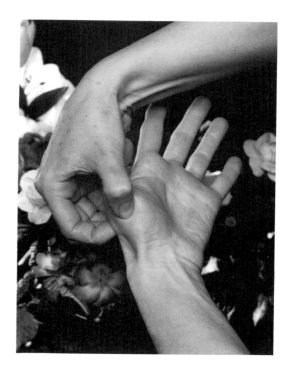

Often, much of spine tension is stored below the
knuckle area of the small finger and in the fleshy
part below the thumb. If there is a particularly sore
spot, use a little more pressure for a few seconds to
see if the pain will release.

For sciatic nerve pain, use your thumbs to gently walk down the inside of the wrist on both sides . .

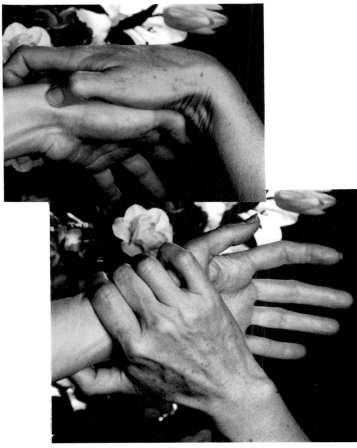

It is important to remember that all reflexology done either by yourself or a reflexologist during your pregnancy should be gentle and comforting. You should only experience minor pain on the reflex points for the pituitary gland, the adrenals, or somewhere you are having problems.

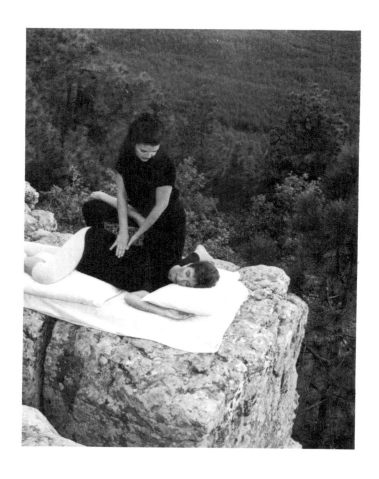

NON-BRUTAL SHIATSU IS GREAT TOO

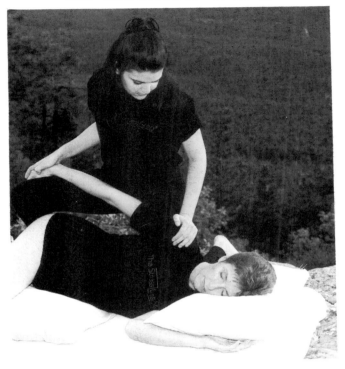

Shiatsu, literally translated as finger pressure, is a type of bodywork that was developed in Japan. It is based on the traditional Chinese philosophy of medicine that has evolved during the past 4000 years. A principle axiom of this philosophy is that a human being is composed of <u>both</u> the physical mass of the body <u>and</u> energy flows. These energy flows are connected to the autonomic nervous

system and the subconscious mind. When your energy
flows freely and evenly your physical body remains
healthy, pain-free and functions efficiently. If energy
becomes blocked or the flows become uneven, physical
pain and sickness result. Uneven energy flows and energy
blocks are created by stress and tension.

Shiatsu follows the same principles of energy flows as
acupuncture. That is, pain and sickness result from energy
blocks or uneven flows along 14 meridians in the body.
These meridians run on the back, front inside and outside
of your body. Each meridian runs on the right and left side
of your body.

Each energy meridian is linked to a physical organ, such
as the heart or liver, and to a body function. Pressure at
various points along these meridians maintains balanced
flows and releases any blocked energy. Shiatsu is also
called acupressure. The amount of pressure used relates
to the condition of your body and its response.

There are two types of shiatsu. I call them the "brutal and
non-brutal" varieties. The non-brutal shiatsu is the variety
where the practitioner is taught to feel your energy flows
and uses only as much pressure as they feel your body
needs. In addition, while one hand applies pressure, the

practitioner's other hand is placed on another part of the meridian or energy flow to balance it . . .

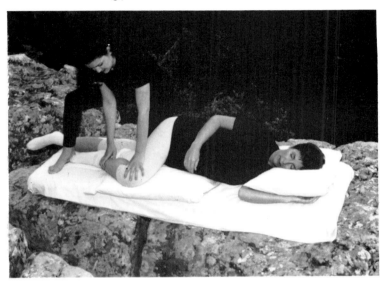

This form of shiatsu is the more sensitive, studious, and methodical variety.

The non-brutal variety was the original form developed in Japan. Other countries have adapted shiatsu and now utilize much harsher approaches. For example, Korean shiatsu can be very aggressive and very harsh. Such an approach is not appropriate for pregnancy.

The Japanese, non-brutal shiatsu is what should be used while you are pregnant. This variety is especially effective for pregnancy. It not only stimulates circulation and lymph drainage, it also relieves pain. For example, it can be used successfully when you're pregnant to reduce back pain caused by your changing posture.

Just like a maternity massage, even non-brutal shiatsu is done very gently during your pregnancy. As one experienced practitioner explained, "I don't intrude as I would in a regular shiatsu session. Instead, I move with the energy . . . I must be much more sensitive and feel where I am able to work and where I shouldn't. I have to let her energy guide me. . . I am more of a passive assistant than the activator in a regular session . . . These pregnancy sessions are so wonderful. It's amazing what happens. When a woman is pregnant, her energy is so powerful, it's like a balloon filling my hand. Finger pressure doesn't match it or relate to it. You just move with this fantastic energy."

The shiatsu practitioner will be watching for the response of your baby as well as the response of your body to their pressure. One shiatsu practitioner pointed out that when she has used too much pressure, it is the baby that responds dramatically. She immediately feels a sudden, strong pulsing energy from the baby. It takes very soothing work to calm the baby if too much pressure is used.

Instead of finger pressure, during pregnancy shiatsu, the practitioner will more often hold the point or stretch the area to release blocked energy . . .

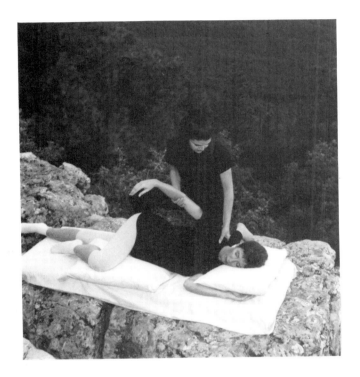

In other cases, the practitioner may hold the point and then move your body to add minimal, but effective pressure. In essence, your own body moves only as much as is necessary to create the pressure needed to release blocked energy and balance the flow. Throughout the session, you will find that the focus of the work will be on stretching and breathing. In addition, more time will be spent on your joints, such as your shoulders and hips.

For a shiatsu session, you should wear either loose fitting clothes or tights that are flexible and comfortable. Just as in a maternity massage, you will be lying on your sides . . .

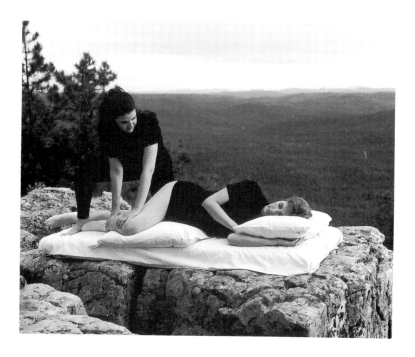

Pillows will be positioned similarly also. That is, one will be placed under your neck and head; another will be put under your leg and your belly.

Sometimes shiatsu can be done while you are sitting, but since lying on your side with pillows puts you in the most relaxing and comfortable position, this is the way it will be done by most shiatsu practitioners. In both positions, all meridians can be easily, gently, and effectively accessed.

The sequence of a shiatsu session depends upon your body and the flow of energy along the 14 meridians. Unlike a typical shiatsu session, minimal work will be done on the hara, the area around the stomach and abdomen. In a maternity session, your shiatsu practitioner will limit work on the hara to sensing your energy flows. If you are or have been nauseous, a little additional work will be done on the stomach meridian to settle your stomach . . .

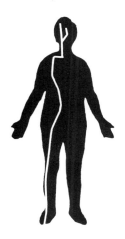

Stomach Meridian

Once this preliminary work is done, you will turn on your
side. When you are comfortable, the shiatsu will generally
begin on the neck and head . . .

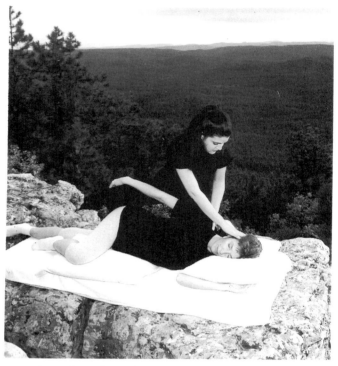

On your head and neck, some additional time may be
spent on the stomach meridian points if you have morning
sickness. Work on other points will primarily help with sinus
congestion and headaches. From your head and neck,
the shiatsu practitioner will proceed along one side of your
body to your shoulders.

The work on your shoulders will primarily be done on the lung and large intestine meridians . . .

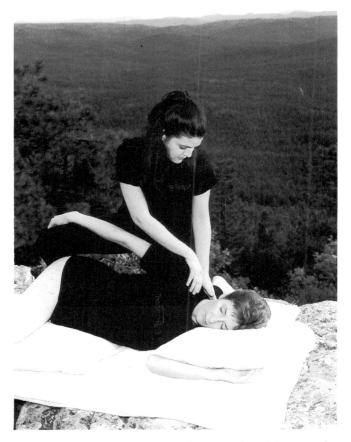

This will help relax the tension in your shoulders and diaphragm. Relaxation of your diaphragm will become more important as your baby grows and puts increasing pressure on it. You will find this work on your shoulders to be very helpful for breathing more easily. The work on your shoulders will include stretching your neck . . .

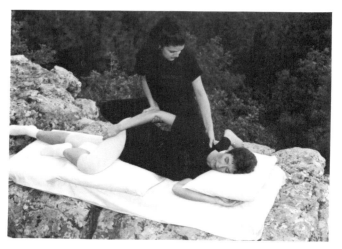

The shiatsu practitioner will also rotate your arm at your shoulder . . .

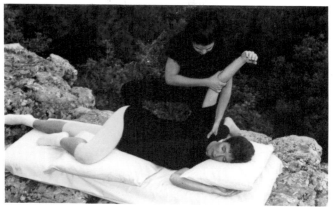

The stretching and rotating of your arm are very effective for releasing blocked energy along meridians in your shoulders and neck. Some gentle pressure may be used to further relax your shoulders and neck. The work on your arms will be primarily on the large intestine meridian. Work on these points can help with headaches, diarrhea, and general well-being. Your lung meridian also runs along your arm. Balancing this meridian will make breathing easier.

When your shoulders feel relaxed, the practitioner will move from your shoulders and arms to your waist and back . . .

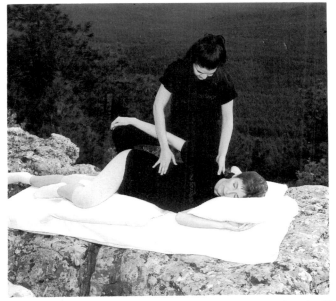

On your back, the primary meridian to be worked will be the bladder meridian. The bladder meridian is particularly important for pregnant women. Working this meridian releases tension in the back, particularly in the lumbar and sacral areas. To effectively work on the bladder meridian, most of the shiatsu will be concentrated on the points along your spine.

As your shiatsu practitioner focuses on your bladder meridian, the work will progress down your hip and leg . . .

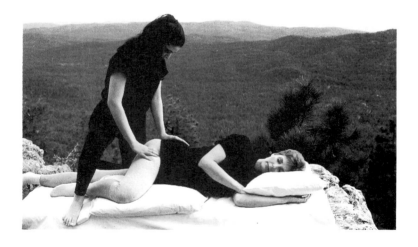

Work done on your hips and legs can be very helpful if you are experiencing poor circulation in your legs. This work will also help general fatigue in your legs.

The shiatsu will continue toward your feet. Some of the important points on the bladder meridian are located around your ankle . . .

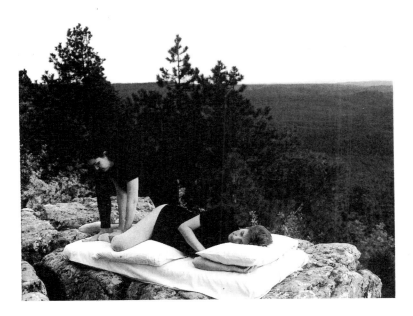

Working the bladder points around the ankle strengthens the entire spine from your sacrum to your neck. These points are also effective for easing a stiff neck, posterior headaches, and burning urination. One point, Bladder 62, located below the tip of your ankle near your Achilles tendon is particularly effective for relieving restlessness and insomnia.

After one side of your body is finished, you will turn over so the other side can be accessed. Because each meridian runs up and down both sides of your body, the work will be similar. It will change only if the energy has shifted sufficiently during the work on the first side.

Besides placing you in the most comfortable position, working on the outer sides of your body also enables your shiatsu practitioner to avoid the meridians not recommended for pregnancy work . . .

1. The spleen meridian.

   The spleen meridian is important because it is one of the two meridians that regulate hormone secretions. It starts near the bottom of the big toe nail and moves along the inside edge of the top of the foot to the ankle. It then progresses along a line up the inside of the calf and thigh muscle to the groin . . .

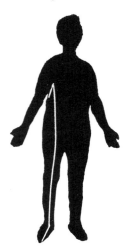

The Spleen Meridian

The spleen meridian goes up the front of your torso to right above your underarm. This meridian then drops on the side of your torso just below your underarm where it ends.

The spleen meridian is also important in Oriental medicine because it is believed to regulate the blood and hemorrhaging. It is considered directly responsible for uterine bleeding. Inappropriate pressure on this meridian can cause uterine contractions and spotting.

The most powerful spleen point is spleen 6, located four fingers above the ankle bone on the inside of the calf. This point is utilized to speed a baby's delivery. It will be discussed more in the chapter "Shiatsu For Labor Ease."

2. The kidney meridian

It is important to work carefully and gently near the kidney meridian because it is believed to also regulate hormone secretion. The kidney meridian begins on the bottom of your foot, between the balls of the big and little toes . . .

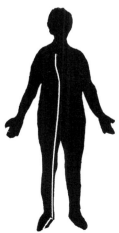

The Kidney Meridian

It then moves around the inside of the ankle and up the inside of the calf and thigh.

Kidney 1 is particularly important to avoid. It is a very powerful point and is located on the sole of the foot, midway across it and just behind the ball of the foot. Inappropriate pressure on this point is avoided because it could move your energy too much instead of maintaining or enhancing the balanced flow which is best for pregnancy. There are several other points on the kidney meridian that will be avoided. They are located on the inside of your foot and leg.

Both the spleen and kidney meridians flow on the <u>inside and front </u>of your legs and torso. The meridians on which work will be done while your are pregnant are located on the <u>outside and back </u>of your legs, arms and torso.

Just as with a maternity massage, there are also some other areas that must be avoided. They are similar to those discussed previously in the section of maternity massage. The areas that will be avoided are. . .

1. Top of the shoulders & near the shoulder blades.

This area contains important points on the gall bladder, small intestine, and bladder meridians. These points are known as release points for the vagina and uterus. Stimulation could cause cramps or premature labor. As you will find out in the chapter *Shiatsu For Labor,* one of these points is very helpful for speeding delivery.

2. Liver 2, 3 & 4

The liver meridian is important for shiatsu when you are pregnant because in Oriental medicine it is believed to regulate the diffusion of your blood. When too much pressure is applied to the liver meridian, your blood is dispersed to your extremities, instead of keeping it concentrated in your placenta where it is most needed by your baby. The important points along your liver meridian are located on your feet. Liver 3 is between your big and second toes, about a half-inch from the junction between these toes. Liver 4 can be found on the top of your foot where your foot and leg join -- slightly below your ankle on the front.

Liver 2 is particularly powerful. It is located at the base of your big toe. This is the point that is stimulated when a woman is not having menstrual periods. Many times her period will begin during a shiatsu session after this point has been worked.

3. Bladder 60

This point is located at the bottom tip of your ankle. Inappropriate pressure on this point will stimulate urination.

There are several other points up the neck related to your gall bladder meridian that should not be worked aggressively. But, if your shiatsu practitioner is sensitive and working with minimal pressure on your neck, the energy flow along the gall bladder meridian will be balanced effectively without unnecessary stimulation.

The important point to remember about shiatsu is that it does work wonders. Because it impacts both the physical mass and energy flows of your body, it is very powerful. I personally turn to shiatsu whenever I am sick. A half-hour of shiatsu when I've had the stomach flu has made me feel as if I had never been sick. I've also found it to be the perfect antidote for headaches and sinus congestion. For the discomforts of pregnancy, there is not much that can equal a shiatsu practitioner who knows how to move with the fantastic energy of you and your baby.

A FEW PRECAUTIONS

As beneficial as maternity massage, shiatsu and reflexology can be, there are a few situations where they are not appropriate. The contraindications for maternity bodywork, that is the situations where maternity bodywork is not advised, include . .

1. Vaginal bleeding or spotting
2. Vaginal discharge
3. Abdominal pains
4. Sudden swelling or edema
5. Fever
6. Excessive protein in the urine
7. Rapid weight gain
8. Blurring vision
9. Decreased fetal movement over a 24-hour period

There are several reasons why maternity bodywork is not recommended if these conditions exist. If you are bleeding, a massage would stimulate the blood flow thus producing more vaginal bleeding or discharge. If a fever is present, there is an indication of an infection and massage or other type of bodywork could stimulate the infection further, thus possibly making the fever rise.

The other conditions could be warning signs of more potential problems. For example, abdominal pains could be a warning of a potential miscarriage or premature labor. Sudden excessive swelling of the legs or hands, which is known as edema, could be a symptom of toxemia, a serious condition or poisoning that occurs during pregnancy.

Additionally, it is best to schedule your massage so that it will not occur immediately after a <u>meal.</u> Try to allow at least two hours after a <u>meal</u> before a massage. This delay is important because stimulating the blood flow will direct it away from the stomach and intestines, where it is needed for proper digestion.

One last point: it is important to consult your doctor before having massage. If your doctor is not knowledgeable about maternity massage, make sure that you have no complications or conditions that would worsen with increased blood flow and lymph drainage. If your doctor believes that there are medical conditions or complications preventing you from having a massage, ask when it would be possible to have one. Also ask if a massage could help alleviate any discomfort caused by the medical condition or complication you are currently experiencing.

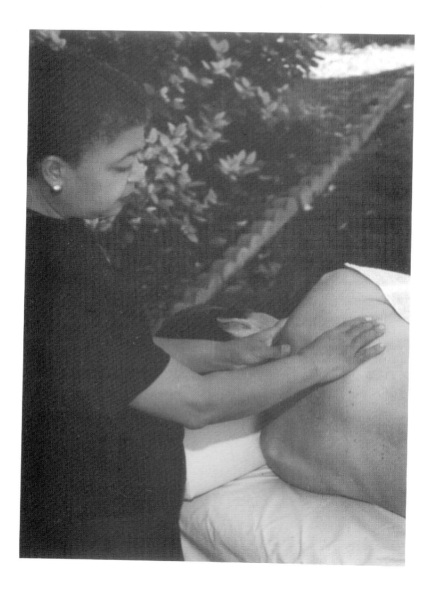

SHIATSU FOR LABOR

Many women have found massage, and especially shiatsu, to be particularly helpful during labor. In 1984, a study was completed that examined the impact of touch during labor. This study, discussed in the November/December 1986 issue of *The Journal of Nurse-Midwifery*, showed that all the women in labor responded positively when touched or massaged.

As preparation for your delivery, you may want to arrange for your massage therapist to be available during your delivery for massage, or you may want your massage therapist to work with your delivery partner to teach him or her how to massage your back and legs during delivery. General massage on your back and legs will provide much relief during labor, and it is easily and quickly taught. For a back massage, you can either lie on your side as you do during a maternity massage or you can sit in a chair and lean forward on the back of the chair with pillows used as needed. Your partner can massage your legs in whatever position you find comfortable.

Massage on your lower back and buttocks can help because relaxing your muscles in your lower back and

buttocks eliminates any muscle tension that may be
blocking or delaying the descent of the baby's head. If
your legs start shaking during the delivery, have someone
massage your inner and upper thighs. Have them stroke
upward and smoothly, keeping the flow as continuous as
possible.

It is also recommended that your delivery partner learn a
few shiatsu points. Recently, more and more midwives
are turning to shiatsu for assistance in alleviating pain,
solving minor problems, and speeding delivery. These
midwives have found that by applying pressure at specific
points on selected meridians, they can have major
positive impact on the delivery process.

There are several points that you or your delivery partner
can access which may be very beneficial for you. During
the early stages of labor, that is, when your contractions
are not that persistent or frequent, it is helpful to press each
point several times for about 10 to 15 seconds each time.
Wait for a while before repeating the pressure. Once you
enter the final stage of labor when your contractions are
only about a minute apart, then pressure on each point
should continue until you feel a change.

Pressure on the following points will help to speed delivery and reduce some of the pain you are experiencing in the final stage of labor . . .

1. Stomach 36

> This point is located at the top of the shin bone, in the curve where the bone widens toward the knee. One way to find this point is to place your hand on your kneecap. Then let your fingers extend around your knee and down your leg. The tip of your fourth finger should be just about on the outside of the shinbone, where this point is located . . .

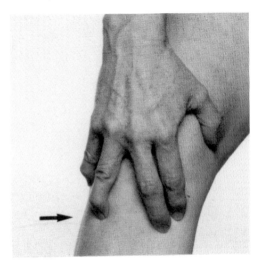

> Have your partner hold this point with their right hand and then have them place their other hand on your shoulder, wherever they feel is appropriate. They should apply pressure on this point until you feel something change.

Pressure on this point should create a strong sensation, extending down to the ankle. It will relieve tension in the legs and help to relax your whole body.

2. Bladder 67

This point is located on the outside of the little toe at the corner of the nail, about 1/8 of an inch from the lower corner of the nail. It is used by experienced shiatsu practitioners to turn babies. It can be utilized by your partner to speed your delivery. Stimulation of this point will bring your energy down to your womb and concentrate it there so that your entire being will be focused on your delivery. It is this concentration which helps to speed your delivery . . .

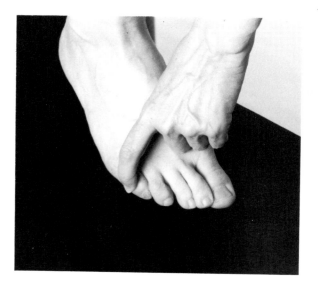

Apply pressure on this point with the tip of your thumb or finger. You can begin to apply pressure to this point a week or so before your expected delivery. Before your labor begins, apply pressure to this point about 10 to 15 seconds three times. Once labor has begun, apply pressure until you feel a change in your body. When applying pressure to this point, your partner should place their balancing hand on your knee or thigh.

3. Bladder 60 and 62

These points are located on your ankle and Achilles tendon. Bladder 60 is located just beside your ankle . . .

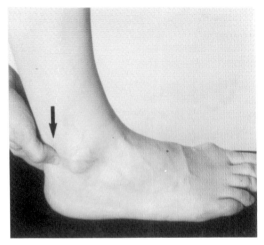

Bladder 62 is located a little below your ankle. Pressure on these points will help relax your leg muscles. They are also effective for relieving restlessness. Stimulation of these points will produce a calming influence. You will find this needed more and more frequently as the final stage of your labor progresses. One benefit of this point is that it is very accessible, not matter what is happening to you.

4. Large Intestine 4

This point is also called "the Great Eliminator." It is located in the middle of the web of flesh between the bones of the thumb and index finger.

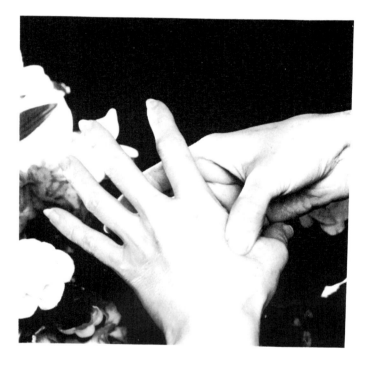

Hold this point with your thumb on one side of your hand and your finger on the other side. Press this point from both sides. Your partner may want to hold your shoulder or elbow while pressing this point.

4. Spleen 6

This area is called the Three Yin Meeting Point. It is considered the most powerful point for speeding delivery because several meridians run through this area, including the spleen and kidney meridians.

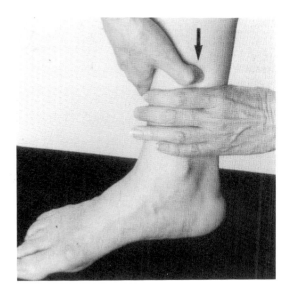

Pressure on this point can stimulate uterine contractions to speed the delivery process. Have your partner hold the inside of your knee or the side of your belly when applying pressure to this point.

5. Gall Bladder 21

You will find this point on your shoulder, slightly on the back side. It is located between the midpoint of the clavicle and the superior border of the scapula. You can find it by tracing a straight line up from your nipple to the top of your shoulder. Or think about the place that a man puts his hand on your shoulder when he wants you to be closer physically with you. All men put their hand on a woman's shoulder in the same place . . .

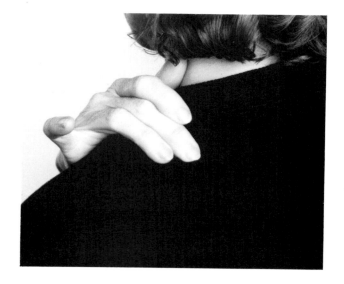

As you begin to bear down during the final stages of labor, have your partner press "Gall Bladder 21" on the top of each shoulder. As with the other points, hold this pressure until you feel changes in your body. The balancing place for your partner's other hand can be on your lower back on the opposite side of your spine.

The gall bladder meridian is concerned with the distribution of energy in your body. By bearing down on Gall Bladder 21, you focus all your body's energy on the delivery process. Pressure on this point can also be used to stimulate breast milk production after your baby is born.

Delivery is a strenuous and painful process no matter what. But, the effort and pain can be reduced with shiatsu. Pressure on certain points can speed delivery and thus shorten the time. Stimulating other points can relieve much of the pain. Learning the location of these points is easy and quick. It's worth the minimal effort required to make your delivery as easy and quick as possible.

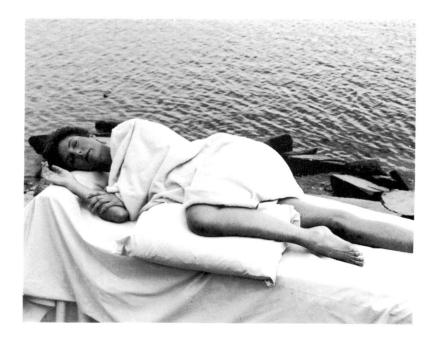

POST- DELIVERY MASSAGE

Just as a maternity massage aids you during pregnancy, a massage within days after the baby is born has many benefits also. Physically, a post-delivery massage can work wonders on the aches and pains from the delivery. Our experience at The Stress Less Step includes many examples of such benefits . . .

> One woman couldn't stand up straight after a C-section - the pain was so intense. The day she arrived home from the hospital, she called for a massage. The massage she was given was the same as that given to her when she was pregnant. At the end, she got off the table and stood tall. All the pain and tension had left her body, and she was ready to go home and take care of her new baby.
>
> Cindy found a massage the only way to cope with the pain from the epidural. As soon as the therapist started massaging her back, she could feel the pain lessen.

Post-delivery massages are beneficial for women who have had C-sections and normal deliveries. Recovery from a C-section is quickened by post-delivery massages. Because the massage stimulates the circulation, the healing process accelerates. In addition, a massage will alleviate much of the pain associated with surgery.

Likewise, massages can relieve the muscle tension and strain resulting from a strenuous delivery - particularly lower back pain. For abdominal discomfort, a post-delivery massage strengthens the body's cleaning action to eliminate anything left over from the placenta and assists the contraction of the uterus.

Massages additionally help you with any depression and irritability after the delivery. An exhaustion and depression like nothing she had ever felt hit Stephanie shortly after the delivery. What a difference from her fantasies of supreme bliss she had expected once her baby was in her arms! She never knew "postpartum blues" could be so blue. If her friend hadn't forced her to use that shower present of a massage, she's not sure what would have happened. She just knows that the massage changed her mood and rejuvenated her.

It is not difficult to understand how a massage can change a woman's mood so quickly. The mood swings following a delivery are the result of the gradual reduction of the thyroid hormone in your body. A post-delivery massage stimulates glandular secretions. This stabilizes hormonal levels thus making their depression-like side effects less severe.

Further, post-delivery massages can help with the sleepless nights of living with a newborn. New mother after new mother has told us how important massages are during those first couple of months. For example, Barbara at first felt a little guilty about leaving her baby for just an hour to get a massage, but she was so tired - and her own mother was watching the baby. She changed her mind as soon as the massage started. What she had expected to be just an hour getaway seemed like a day of relief and she needed every minute of it. Post-delivery massages are particularly effective to cope with sleepless nights. Remember: a relaxing massage is the equivalent of 4 hours of sleep. The increased circulation of the massage minimizes physical fatigue by bringing more oxygen to the blood stream and cells.

Post-delivery massage also sedates the nervous system. This sedation alleviates headaches and lower back pain so that when time is available for a nap, it can quickly and easily be enjoyed. As we all know, a mother of a newborn needs all the energy and stamina she can get.

Post-delivery massage can also help with breast-milk production. Massage stimulates the mammary glands in the breast area. The stimulation of these glands helps produce more milk.

Lastly, massage can effectively eliminate the muscle strain you will experience in your shoulders from holding your baby. This strain is caused by constantly holding and carrying your baby on your shoulder or in your arms -- a strenuous exercise for everyone's shoulder muscles, no matter what condition you are in. You will also notice a new muscle strain when you are breast-feeding your baby. Holding your baby as you breast feed is another new position and exercise for your shoulder and arm muscles. As your baby gains weight, the muscle strain travels to your lower back when you use your entire upper body to support this weight. This new muscle strain and pain occurs with all new mothers. It builds day by day and week by week. Massages during this new exertion by your shoulder muscles can stop the build-up of tension and therefore the increasing level of pain. Massages can be particularly effective for those prolonged exertions of your shoulder and back muscles. There is nothing that can produce shoulder and back pain so quickly as holding a sick or upset baby for hour after hour. A massage after such an episode is just what is needed. The muscle tension is quickly released and the pain in relieved.

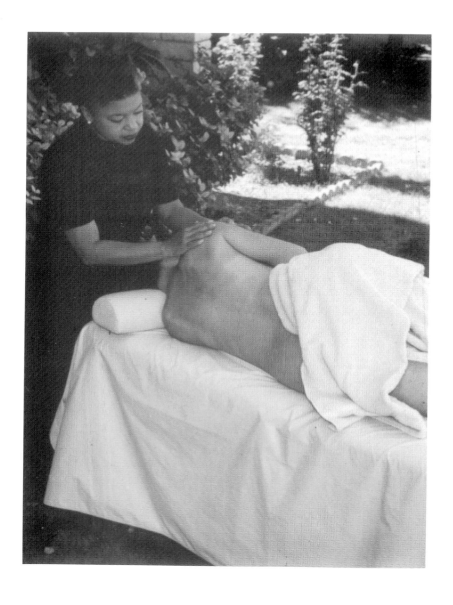

FINDING A MATERNITY MASSAGE

There are several approaches which can help you find a massage therapist who is qualified to give a maternity massage that is just right for you. First, you can ask your doctor for referrals. If your doctor is not aware of someone, ask friends and acquaintances. Or, talk with local chiropractors, your favorite beautician and the concierge of the best local hotel. The first places a massage therapist will contact to build business include chiropractors, beauty salons, and local hotels.

Once you have the names of several candidates, interview them yourself. If you have been referred to a massage facility, request information about the massage therapists who do the maternity massages. Good questions to ask relate to . . .

- Years of experience with maternity massage
- Frequency of doing maternity massage

You can also ask about training in maternity massage, but you should remember that official training for maternity massage is a very new phenomena. Courses in maternity massage have only been offered during the past 3 or 4 years. A massage therapist with many years of experience in maternity massage is the best choice.

The most important questions to ask relate to the approach of the massage therapist to maternity massage. Ask how a maternity massage differs from a regular massage. Now that you know what to expect, you know what they should say. If you aren't told the differences discussed before, you know the person is not sufficiently trained for your maternity massage.

Don't be afraid to ask questions about whether or not the facilities are comfortable for a pregnant woman. Are massage rooms private? Many spas perform massages in open areas. Are dressing rooms sufficiently large for you to undress and dress in the final trimester with ease? Can you easily and quickly move from the massage table to a bathroom? One very attractive feature for a facility providing maternity massage is somewhere to sleep comfortably for several hours after the massage. Many pregnant women find the peace and relaxation of a massage just what is needed to finally fall into a deep sleep. It is much easier to rest if there is somewhere close by for a quick nap.

You can ask about pregnancy massage tables also, but
don't expect to find them. They are a very recent
invention, and questions have already been raised about
the appropriateness and comfort of these tables. The key
to comfort during a maternity massage is to minimize the
strain of the baby's weight on the mother's back, stomach,
shoulders and legs. In addition, there should be no
physical pressure placed on the baby.

With a maternity massage table, you eventually lie on
your stomach, with a hole cut in the table for your
stomach and some type of support provided below for
the belly. Most practitioners of maternity massage
believe that this table <u>adds</u> to the strain on the woman's
back, and places too much pressure on the breasts and
thighs. There is no way when a pregnant woman is lying on
her stomach that some type of pressure won't be placed
on the areas supporting her. Either the pressure will occur
somewhere on the chest or on the thighs. Most
practitioners of maternity massage believe that placing a
woman on her side is the only way to access a woman's
back for massage without creating unnecessary pressure.
They have found that it is much more effective and
comfortable. "With enough pillows, you can relax <u>every</u>
muscle and still massage all the muscles correctly."

Lastly, if the facility or spa you visit has a sauna, whirlpool, Jacuzzi, hot tub, hot bath or steam room, <u>don't use them.</u> Anything that rapidly raises your body temperature is dangerous for your baby. Caution should also be used with bodywraps. Although some bodywraps can assist your pregnancy by helping your body rid itself of toxins and excessive water retention, any that accomplish this with heat or sweating is not good for your pregnancy. Select <u>only</u> those bodywraps which utilize <u>no</u> additional heat and produce <u>no</u> sweating or temperature increases

A FEW DO'S AND DON'TS

There are few more points for you to remember as you begin to experience the wonders of maternity massages . . .

1. Do tell your massage therapist as soon as you start trying to conceive.

   Telling your massage therapist early can help you in several ways. First, by stimulating certain areas, you may be able to enhance your fertility. It is possible to lengthen the 24-hour period when a woman is most fertile. Most important, women are more likely to conceive when they are relaxed and peaceful.

   Second, if you do conceive, the massage therapist will have already changed the massage so that it won't encourage a miscarriage.

2. Don't worry about how you will look during your massage.

   Many women become embarrassed as they gain weight and their shape changes. And they wonder about what a massage therapist will think when they see everything. First, you must remember that your massage therapist will actually see very little of you. Yes, they will see your legs and they will see your arms and back, but you are never put in a position where they visually examine your body. And, they generally will be striving to provide you as much modesty as possible.

Additionally, you should realize that a massage therapist's thoughts are not on an evaluation of your body. A massage therapist is thinking about locating problems. While they are giving a massage, they are watching your muscles respond to their strength and technique. They are also concentrating on following the lines of your muscles. They really are not as aware as you would think of how you look as a person.

Remember also that all persons getting massage are lying flat on a table, not in a particularly flattering position. In fact, no one looks that attractive while getting a massage. Your muscles are being pulled in many directions and everything sags. You may not have realized that photo shoots of massage are staged. Shooting actual massages generally is a waste of time because it is very difficult to obtain an attractive picture of someone getting a massage. Because no one looks that good during a massage, massage therapist don't look. They concentrate on what they are doing, not whether or not you look attractive.

3. Don't wear underwear.

Many women keep some underwear on for the sake of modesty. Unfortunately, underwear generally covers parts of muscles that must be worked to release the total muscle. Underwear also crosses muscles. When you wear underwear, the massage therapist cannot follow the line of your muscles. They must stop the movement before it is completed. This incomplete movement lessens the impact of what they are doing.

4. Do demand to be covered adequately.

You should be covered adequately to maintain your body's warmth. As your body relaxes, your body's temperature drops. Once you become uncomfortably cool, your muscles begin to tense and tighten. You should be covered so that as your body relaxes, your temperature does not drop too much.

Also important, it is necessary that the correct level of professionalism be shown. You should not feel exposed in any way. The only area of you which your massage therapist should be able to see is the one they are working on, e.g. your leg, your arm or your back.

5. Do speak up immediately if you have <u>any</u> discomfort during the massage.

If you experience discomfort, it is a sign that what the massage therapist is doing is not appropriate for you. It is not necessary that you explain what is wrong or why. What's important is that you let your massage therapist know that what is being done does not feel good.

In massage, there are many techniques and strokes that can be used -- somewhat like a bag of tricks. If one isn't right for you, there are plenty more. Your speaking up is not a criticism of your massage therapist. This information is what is needed to find the best techniques, pressure, tempo, and flow for you and your baby.

Research has shown that when you feel pain, your heart rate and blood pressure increase rapidly. Since your baby needs a stable, peaceful environment, such dramatic changes are not desirable. More important, pain is a way for your body to tell you something is wrong. Whenever you feel pain during a maternity massage, speak up immediately.

6. Do tell your massage therapist how your body responded to your prior massage.

In fact, you should expect your massage therapist to ask you how you felt after the last massage. This information will tell a massage therapist if adjustments are needed. She or he will be looking for any techniques or areas that produced subsequent discomfort for you and your baby. Your massage therapist wants to know what works best for you and how your pregnancy is progressing.

7. Don't talk during the massage except when you have any discomfort.

A good massage requires intense concentration from your massage therapist. This is needed to achieve and maintain the sensitivity required to feel how your body responds to a gentle massage. It is this concentration that also produces the insight as to what is best for you and your baby.

If you try to direct the massage or constantly interrupt your massage therapist, she or he will stop the flow of the massage movement, stroke or technique.

When you stop the movement, you limit its beneficial impact. It becomes an unfinished stroke or technique, not the complete approach that is needed for its true effectiveness.

You should only speak up if you are uncomfortable. Otherwise, let your massage therapist do their job. If you want to talk with them, schedule extra time before or after the massage.

8. Do stop the massage if the therapist uses a single finger or knuckles, or digs into your muscles, or works incorrectly on problematic areas.

   The potential for this occurring should be low if you have screened the massage therapist for expertise in maternity massage, but you may encounter someone with outstanding references who really doesn't know what they are doing during a maternity massage. If a massage therapist uses her knuckles or works too deeply, you know they are not for you. Stop the massage immediately and find someone else. Don't worry about upsetting the massage therapist, you and your baby are too important.

   If you have had good massages from this person before, it is also important to stop the massage. Not often, but sometimes, a massage therapist's mind wanders. If this happens, it is a sign for you that this is not the time for this person to be giving a maternity massage.

9. Don't ask for a strong massage.

There are many superstitions about saying "no" to a pregnant woman. One of the major conflicts facing massage therapist is doing the massage they know is best for a pregnant woman when the woman is telling them to go stronger or spend more time on prohibited areas. It is best to show some patience. Let them use their expertise. Just wait and see what happens. Most women are shocked that a gentle massage with all the time spent in the "wrong" areas can alleviate so much pain and discomfort.

10. Do feel free to ask your massage therapist questions.

When a massage therapist works with pregnant women for any length of time, they become privy to many women facing the same situations, fears, discomforts, sensations, and new experiences. They can share their insights as to what has helped other women and what hasn't.

The most important thing to remember about maternity massage is that a healthy pregnancy is a <u>peaceful</u> pregnancy. Maternity massage can help you develop and maintain the physical and mental peace that is necessary for a healthy pregnancy. It can also take away almost all of the discomforts so you can totally enjoy this unique and wondrous experience.

CONCLUSION

Being pregnant is one of the most special experiences you will ever have. It's important that you enjoy your pregnancy and your new baby as much as possible. If massage or other types of bodywork can relieve the discomforts and put you in the best frame of mind for this unique time, there's no reason to wait. You will see that the results will be wonderful. More important, with maternity massage, you can focus on the miracle before you. I can't recommend it too highly.

The key to successfully obtaining maternity massage is to be an educated buyer. The goal of this book is to give you the information you need. So now that you've read it, there's nothing to stop you from finding relief and peace of mind for a healthy and happy pregnancy.

Lastly, you don't have to stop getting massages after your baby is no longer a baby. Many women find massages a necessity for the additional back strain that comes from lifting and carrying a child for the next two years or more. Not only is massage a great pain reliever, it's the only healthy indulgence I know.

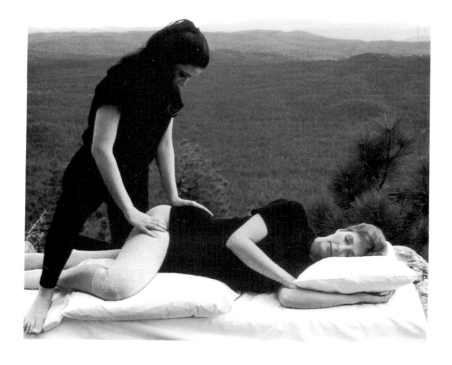

GLOSSARY

Adrenal Gland: A triangular gland covering the top of each kidney. The secretions of these glands influence blood flow, heart rates, glucose production, and digestion. These glands are very sensitive to your emotional state.

Amniocentesis: The puncture of the amniotic sac using a needle to obtain amniotic fluid. This fluid is then tested for genetic and biochemical disorders.

Anemia: A condition where the number of red blood cells is less than required to provide sufficient oxygen for your body. Symptoms include pale skin, fatigue and weakness, general malaise, depression, and headaches.

Autonomic Nervous System: The part of your nervous system that is concerned with the control of the involuntary functions of your body, such as your blood pressure and heart beat. It works "automatically," that is without your conscious action. This system also regulates glands such as your salivary, gastric and sweat glands.

Diaphragm: The muscular wall that separates the abdomen from your chest. It relaxes each time you exhale and it contracts each time you inhale. It permits and/or restricts the descent of your lungs as you breath.

Edema: A condition where your body's tissues contain excessive amounts of tissue fluid. There are many causes of edema, such as consumption of excess salt or the decreased atmospheric pressure you experience when you fly. It can be a mild condition where bedrest is sufficient to relieve it, or it can more serious.

Endocrinological Balance: A balance of your ductless glandular system whose secretions are discharged into your blood and lymph. The glands include the pituitary, thyroid, parathyroid, and adrenal glands. The ovaries and testes are also included in this system.

Endorphins: Chemical substances produced in the brain that function like morphine, tranquilizers or opiates. They are synthesized in the pituitary gland. They are important for pain relief, sedation, and behavior control. Stimulation of endorphin production can produce peacefulness, mental stress reduction and tranquillity.

Enkephalins: Chemical substances produced in the brain that act as tranquilizers or opiates. They differ from endorphins because they can suppress "Substance P" which is very important in our sense of pain. Enkephalins are responsible for increasing your threshold for pain dramatically. Acupuncture or other influences on Oriental energy points are believed to release enkephalins into your cerebral-spinal fluid.

Homeostasis: The state of dynamic equilibrium of your internal body.

Lactic Acid: A liquid that is formed during muscular activity.

Lymph: The fluid formed in tissue spaces throughout your body. When lymph flows through lymph nodes, it is cleansed of foreign matters, such as bacteria and toxins.

Lymphatic System: The system that is responsible for moving lymph from tissues to your bloodstream. It includes lymph capillaries, nodes, vessels and ducts. It is the primary cleansing system of your body.

Melanin: The pigment that is responsible for the color of your hair and skin.

Occipital: The area in the back part of your head, at the base of your skull.

Pituitary Gland: A small gland connected to the base of your brain. It secretes a number of hormones that regulate your body's processes, including growth, reproduction, and metabolism.

Receptors: A component of a cell that combines with a drug, hormone, chemical, or other mediator to change the function of a cell. They are classified by the nature of the stimuli. Sensory receptors are nerve-endings responding to stimuli from outside your body such as touch and temperature.

Sacrum: The triangular bone situated at the base of your spine.

Sciatic Nerve: The largest nerve in your body. It begins in your pelvis and runs down the back of your thigh.

Thymus Gland: An organ located just above the heart. It is important for the effective functioning of your immune system.

Thyroid Gland: A gland located in the base of your neck. It has two lobes that can be found on each side of your larynx. Secretions from your thyroid gland influence the overall state of your body. Excessive secretions can prompt restlessness, irritability and hot flashes.

Toxemia: A condition where poisonous products of bacteria are growing in excess in your body. Symptoms include edema, fever, diarrhea, vomiting, and a quickened pulse or breathing.

Toxin: A harmful substance, such as bacteria.

Varicose Veins: Enlarged or twisted veins. They can be caused by impeded circulation.

INDEX

ABOUT THE AUTHOR

Connie A. Cox is the founder and President of The Stress Less Step in New York City, the largest massage/bodywork center in the United States. Living in fast-paced Manhattan, Ms. Cox, a Harvard MBA, saw the need to escape from the stress of everyday life, and would relieve her own tensions with massage. Ms. Cox believes that massage, once regarded primarily as a pampering treatment for the rich, is needed by people from every walk of life. After eight years, Ms. Cox has built The Stress Less Step into a million-dollar enterprise. And her vision has extended West. She recently opened a second center in Scottsdale, Arizona.

Prior to The Stress Less Step, Ms. Cox was a successful banker, corporate planner and business consultant for companies such as Citibank, General Foods and McKinsey & Company. Her expertise: identifying new business opportunities, strategic planning and marketing.

As a business executive, Ms. Cox published numerous articles on strategic planning and marketing. She is also the author of *Selling Information to U.S. Businesses*, the first published documentation of the business information industry in the U.S. *Maternity Massage* is her first book written for the general public.

THE EXPERTS

Hilda Franco (The Pictured Maternity Massage Therapist)

Ms. Franco has been doing massage for over 30 years. Her formal training was obtained at The Swedish Institute. She graduated in June, 1963. Ms. Franco became a New York State licensed massage therapist in 1968. Since that time, she has worked as a massage therapist at massage centers in New York, Puerto Rico, and Arizona. Ms. Franco was not only the person giving Connie Cox massages before she opened The Stress Less Step, she was also the massage therapist who was responsible for suggesting to Ms. Cox that she establish a massage center. Ms. Franco joined The Stress Less Step when it opened in June, 1983. Her responsibilities included screening massage therapist applicants, training newly hired therapists, and teaching maternity massage. In 1993, Ms. Franco became the manager of The Stress Less Step in Scottsdale, Arizona.

Her original knowledge of maternity massage dates back to the early 1970's. At that time, she was taught maternity massage from a licensed massage therapist in Puerto Rico. In the 1970's, there was no formal education in maternity massage at massage schools; the only source of such information came from experienced massage therapists. Since that time her knowledge has been expanded from her own experience with patients. During the past twenty years, she has worked with over 100 pregnant women each year. She has also studied shiatsu for pregnancy. Today, Ms. Franco is one of the few massage therapists in the United States with extensive knowledge and experience regarding maternity massage.

Ofra Naim (The Pictured Shiatsu Practitioner)

Ms. Naim is a practitioner of shiatsu and reflexology. She received her formal training in shiatsu from The Ohashi Institute from 1990 to 1992. She was taught reflexology by Ms. Simone Carbonel. She joined The Stress Less Step in 1993.

Ms. Naim's initial work with pregnancy occurred with a friend who was pregnant. After that experience, she began to study shiatsu for pregnancy from The Ohashi Institute.

THE EXPERTS - CONT.

Dr. Rostilav Tourtchaninov

Dr. Rostilav Tourchaninov is a highly respected orthopedic surgeon from the Ukraine. He was one of the youngest graduates from medical school in Russian, completing the six-year program of the Odessa Medical Institute and earning his degree with honors at the age of 22. He then entered the Kiev Scientific and Research Institute of Orthopedy, where he completed two additional years of specialization in orthopedics. He continued to work as a surgeon at the Kiev Institute until coming to the U.S. in 1991.

Dr. Rostilav Tourtchaninov is one of the few doctors with extensive knowledge of massage therapy. Although Dr. Tourtchaninov was an orthopedic surgeon in the Ukraine, he worked first hand with massage therapy. In Russia and the Ukraine, because medical supplies are extremely scarce and technology is almost nonexistent, surgeons use every alternative possible before and after surgery. As Mr. Tourtchaninov so clearly explains, "When I went into an operating room at the Kiev Scientific and Research Institute of Orthopedy, one of the finest medical centers in Russian, I went in with just my hands and my knife. Most times, there were no anesthetics, no metal pins . . . just my hands and my knife." The result is that as a surgeon, Dr. Tourtchaninov was also trained in many alternative medical approaches such as European chiropractic, acupuncture with electricity, Chinese medicine, nutrition, and massage therapy. At the Kiev Institute, Dr. Tourtchaninov had a staff of massage therapists working for him. He worked with this team to develop effective therapies so that surgery could be avoided. He also directed them in massage therapy required after surgery to insure the patient would regain complete recovery. It was during these years of working with his staff that Dr. Tourtchaninov developed his ability to determine precisely what massage therapy could help and which techniques were most effective.

Dr. Tourchaninov brought his family to the U.S. in 1991 to escape the dangers associated with the nuclear accidents in Chernobyl, located only 100 miles from his home in Kiev. He decided to build a new life in the U.S. so that he could learn and use the latest technology and medical suppliers available in orthopedic surgery. He is presently studying for the medical board exams he must pass to become a licensed surgeon in the U.S.

THE EXPERTS - CONT.

Simone Carbone

Ms. Carbone has been involved with bodywork since 1980 when she began studying foot reflexology, shiatsu, and Ayurvedic medicine in Italy. In 1984, when she came to the United States, she continued her education in these fields by studying with Laura Norman and Martin Ravinsky in New York City. She also entered The Ohashi Institute to further expand her knowledge of shiatsu and to also learn about Jin Shin Do and craniosacral therapy. During the past 8 years, she has been teaching reflexology and shiatsu in a program for continuing education in Rome, Italy. She has also been a teacher of shiatsu at The Ohashi Institute in New York City.

Her first experience with shiatsu and reflexology for pregnancy occurred in 1987 when she worked with a pregnant friend. She worked with her throughout her pregnancy and assisted her in a home delivery. Since that time, she has continued to work with pregnant women; working with them during the pregnancy, assisting with home deliveries, and continuing her help "post partum."

Leslie DeNunzio

Ms. DeNunzio's introduction to massage came while she trained 10 years to become a classical ballet dancer. She began receiving massages on a regular basis as a teenager to battle the tendon problems of dancers. She discovered at that very young age that she was able to perform better and recover faster with weekly massages. She began studying anatomy at the age of 16 when she received a full 4-year scholarship to college in New York City. Her knowledge of anatomy and the beneficial impact of massage was enhanced by her own running program begun after graduation. She entered her first marathon in 1988 and continues to run 60 miles a week.

It was during her training as a runner that she decided to train as a massage therapist. She received her New York State license for massage therapy in 1991 and began working at The Stress Less Step. She was trained in maternity massage by Hilda Franco. She has also taken a course in maternity massage offered by The Swedish Institute. But, it is Ms. Franco's initial training and her own experience that has created the critical knowledge she has about maternity massage. In just the past two years at The Stress Less Step, Ms. DeNunzio has given over 3000 massages, about 20 percent of which were for pregnant women.

THE EXPERTS - CONT.

Geraldine Kelly

Ms. Kelly entered the massage field in 1988 when she attended the Brighton College of Technology in the south of England. At this school, Ms. Kelly studied both massage therapy and aesthetics, but she excelled in massage therapy, receiving "Distinction" in this field. Prior to coming to the U.S., Ms. Kelly worked as a massage therapist in England for several years.

She joined The Stress Less Step in 1992 and was initially taught maternity massage techniques by Hilda Franco. It was Ms. Franco's determination that Ms. Kelly had the appropriate touch, demeanor, and massage knowledge for maternity massages. During the past two years, her knowledge of maternity massage has come primarily from completing about 5 to 7 maternity massages each week.

Marilyn Lavender

Ms. Lavender became interested in bodywork and herbology during her own pregnancy in 1988. The massage therapist giving her massages during the post-partum stage suggested to Ms. Lavender that she study reflexology. Ms. Lavender studied reflexology at The Laura Norman Institute of Reflexology in New York City during 1990 and 1991.

During the past two years, she has worked with numerous pregnant women. She has found reflexology to be particularly helpful during post partum. Once the bleeding has stopped, reflexology helps balance the hormones and establish a balanced, grounded energy level.

THE EXPERTS - CONT.

Rebecca Scott

Ms. Scott started her massage training in 1983 when she took courses in reflexology and shiatsu. This was followed by additional courses in reflexology and Reiki. Ms. Scott received her formal training in Swedish massage therapy in 1985. Her initial interest in bodywork focused on infant massage; Ms. Scott was a nanny and found massage to be very effective for newborns and ill children. After obtaining her NYS massage license, she worked as a massage therapist in a medical clinic for AIDS patients, several health clubs and facial salons. It was during these years that she refined her knowledge of massage. She also took courses in deep-tissue massage and Jin Shin Do.

She began doing maternity massage after taking a course in pregnancy shiatsu at The Ohasi Institute in 1987. She followed this with a pregnancy massage course in 1991 in California. Ms. Scott began working at The Stress Less Step in 1993.

Pieter Sommen

Mr. Sommen's introduction to massage came when he was studying dance. He decided to formally study massage in 1989 and entered The Swedish Institute in New York City. He followed his studies in Swedish massage with shiatsu training both at The Swedish Institute and The Ohasi Institute. In the past three years, his focus has turned to Oriental medicine. He is continuing studies in this field while working at The Stress Less Step and teaching shiatsu at The Swedish Institute.

Mr. Sommen joined The Stress Less Step in 1991. Not only is Mr. Sommen an accomplished practitioner of massage and shiatsu, he is now responsible for screening candidates for massage and shiatsu at The Stress Less Step in New York City.

Renata Stachowicz-Cebula

Ms. Stachowicz-Cebula's initial massage training was obtained while she studied at the Zabrze Medical Vocational College in Poland. During her two years of study there, she was taught many different kinds of physical therapy, including medical massage, kinesiotherapy, Balneother, hydrotherapy, and physiotherapy. This program also included hospital training in orthopedic trauma, neurology, rheumatology, pediatrics, and gynecology.

She was taught maternity massage during her 96 hours of training in the gynecology practice's labor school. This school presented exercise and massage therapy for pregnancy, labor, and post partum. The massage techniques were used in the hospital to help lessen the discomfort of pregnancy and reduce the stress of staying in a hospital for women with high risk pregnancies. With patients with high risk pregnancies, the massages were limited to 10 to 15 minutes. After the maternity massage training, Ms. Stachowicz-Cebula was introduced to infant massage, "the Shantal method."

When Ms. Stachowicz-Cebula completed her physical therapy training, she became a physical therapist in the Gorka Children's Hospital, where she primarily used massage therapy with children with cerebral palsy and other congenital defects. She also taught massage on a part-time basis at Gorka Medical Vocational College.

Ms. Stachowicz-Cebula joined The Stress Less Step in 1988. During the past 6 years, she has given approximately 10 to 12 maternity massages each month. She became more convinced than ever of the benefits during her own pregnancy in 1989. Her co-workers continually gave her massages as she continued to do massage therapy until three days before her son was born. She says that the maternity massages she received helped her understand very clearly the needs and necessities of pregnant women, and how massage techniques specifically impact pregnancies.

Stress Less Publishing, Inc.

7000 East Camelback Road, Scottsdale, AZ 85251

(800) 794-7066

Please send me _____ copies of *Maternity Massage*, at $12.95 each. I have enclosed $_____. (Add $2.75 postage and handling for the first book, and $1.25 for each additional copy. Please send check, money order, or credit card information below. No COD's. Please allow two weeks for delivery.

Name:_____

Street   Address: _____

City:_____State:_____Zip:_____

Charge to my:

Visa   MasterCard   Diners   Discover

Account   No.:_____
Expiration Date:_____

Signature:_____

TO ORDER TOLL FREE: (800) 794-7066
When ordering by phone, please have your credit card information ready.

Quantity discounts available on orders exceeding 5 copies.
Prices subject to change without notice.

Thank you Dan! !

This book was a

great help.

Mar 2002   Sharon